# To Wake In Tears

## Understanding Interstitial Cystitis

### CATHERINE M. SIMONE

### a.k.a. CATH767

IC Hope, Ltd.
Cleveland, Ohio

To Wake In Tears
Understanding Interstitial Cystitis

Copyright © 1998

IC Hope, Ltd.
First Printing 1998

ISBN   0-9667750-0-7

Library of Congress Catalog Card Number
98-74050  CIP

Printed in the United States by Morris Publishing
3212 East Highway 30
Kearney,  NE  68847
1-800-650-7888

For the loving way he dispelled his wisdom,
for his ever-present support and unconditional love,
for his faith in me always...
This book is dedicated with abundant love and respect to my
father...Joseph Michael Simone
...who lived his life with courage, love, and laughter...
and gave to his children the same...

# Acknowledgments

I really want to thank my husband Charlie most of all. To say that you were there for me is nowhere near enough. To explain how your physical presence gave me strength or how you physically took care of me every day. To say that you believed me right from the start...when everyone else was in doubt. To describe how you loved and adored me...with your eyes and through your touch...as if I were a beautiful, healthy princess...not a blob of pain that could no longer care for herself. To thank you for continuously making me laugh even though we were living hell. To try to write it all here is to make light of what you have done for me. My life, my recovery, this book...none would have been possible without you. I'm everything I am because you loved me.

I want to thank my friend and sister-in-law Sue for being there for me right from the start. For all the times you called to check on me and all the times you listened to me complain. For your compassion and concern, I want to thank you. And a special thank you to the rest of Charlie's family for accepting me as I was (with IC) without knowing if I would ever be the healthy wife that I'm sure they wished for their brother and son.

I also want to thank my mom for hanging in there with me, as I most certainly took out most of my anger on her. And my brothers, Mike, Steve, and Lee, thank you for always loving me no matter what. And I want to thank Linda, my friend of 27 years, not only for helping me edit this book, but, as always, for being my true friend.

Many thanks to Cynthia Hart for her insights and guidance, her friendship and love. For the times you were there for me, lifting me out of the pain and showing me the way, I want to thank you. I also want to thank Latifa McNeill, Ernie, and Roland for the insights they provided and the healings they facilitated.

Thank you to my IC friends on line...without whom I would not have found any direction or any hope. A special thank you to Nancy Michelli for starting the IC support group on America On Line. For reaching out and making me feel welcome and then inviting me to be a co-leader (even when I still felt like a "newbie") so that I could give back to others the support and encouragement I got from her. Thank you to Suzanne Bernhardt for all the work you put into compiling the survey in the Appendix and for allowing me to share it in this book. Thank you to Barb Willis, my friend and co-leader of the past 3 years. Thank you for supporting and encouraging me to write this book. And thank you for manning the boards while I was "missing in action".

Thank you to Dr. Thomas Mandat for restoring some of my faith in the medical community and for being the first doctor to treat me in a humane manner since I first got sick. Thank you to Dr. Paul Fugazzotto for his sincere kindness and for the hope he provided me when I so desperately needed it. A special thank you to my friend, Dr. Sherri, for her open mind and her use and modifications of NAET. And thank you to Dr. Joseph Obermeier for his patience and compassion.

Thank you to Joywings, Many Feathers, Soft Paws, and the Little Man.

Thank you to God for all my miracles.

# Preface

CATH767 is my screen name on America On Line. For the past three years or so, I have been mostly housebound, and very often bedridden, with IC and the effects of IC. During this time of seclusion, I have been known to the "world" as CATH767. I was fortunate enough to own a computer when I first got sick. Being able to "speak" with other IC patients on-line was vital to my healing and to my sanity. The computer was my lifeline to the world. At a time when so many people are questioning the effects of the Internet on mankind, this is certainly one if its' stronger benefits. The fact that we have access to the most current medical research and that we can "speak" with people from all across the country...all over the world even...is amazing. We can become aware of the most up to date medical information and browse the medical libraries of famous universities. We are no longer bound by the medical information of one or two doctors who may or may not have the time or interest in researching IC. Very often I have found that IC patients know more about IC than their healthcare providers. We research more. We have the time. We have the desperation and drive to learn as much as we can so that we can get well. The computer offers us thousands of experiences of individuals from all over the world to compare and contrast and learn from. We are able to have choices. We are able to have hope.

# Disclaimer

In this day and age with everybody suing everybody else, books such as these require a disclaimer. I won't say the old standby "check with your doctor before trying any new treatment" because it goes against several points I try to make in this book. But I will say this. Don't do what I did just because I did it. Don't do what I say just because I said it. Look to your own situation, your own experience and your own body, for the answers. Follow your best judgment after learning as much as you possibly can from as many sources as you can. There are so many controversial issues when it comes to this disease, that if everyone had to worry about getting sued, no one would ever say anything. Actually I think that's basically what has happened. The same things seem to be said over and over again in every IC article that I've ever seen. It's difficult to come out and say what you really think for fear of getting sued. I tried not to worry about that as I wrote this book. I prefer to have the information out there, for someone to speak up about this awful disease. As a patient, that is what I would have wanted. And so that is what I try to do here. So please don't sue me.

# Introduction

Imagine waking up in the morning to sharp, stabbing pains in your bladder. Your pelvic area is inflamed as though you ate half a basketball. You try to move to get out of bed and every bone, every muscle in your body, aches. You walk hunched over in agony to the bathroom and hold on to the sink for balance to sit down on the toilet. Your bladder is full, but nothing will come out. The pain increases. Minutes pass and maybe you squeeze out a few drops of burning hot urine. It may take twenty minutes before you can empty your bladder and when you finally get up, you instantly feel like you have to go again. There is no relief. Imagine having to urinate an average of 75 times a day. You fall asleep only out of exhaustion and are constantly awakened by the pain and constant trips to the bathroom. Imagine ground glass in your bladder or maybe a small forest fire. There is blood in your urine and you have an ever-present, constant need to urinate urgently.

Now...you go to the doctor and the nightmare begins. They tell you that nothing is physically wrong with you. Your culture is not showing an infection. You explain to them as best you can that you are not crazy and that the pain and swelling are real. And after all...they can SEE the blood. You beg for their help. You don't know what's wrong with you and you're scared. You ask for something for the pain and they tell you "no, because there's nothing really wrong with you", or "no, we just can't hand out pain medication to anyone who asks for it", or "no, not until we figure out exactly what's wrong with you". And they send you home. But you're still in pain, still bleeding, still in the bathroom every five minutes, and definitely still scared. So you go to a different doctor...this one is the Head of Urology at a prestigious hospital. This one tells you that it is not unusual for women your age to have emotional problems that affect their bladder. "You will just have to learn to live with it," he tells you. You leave his office in tears. Knowing that you don't have emotional problems and that your pain is real, you go to yet another doctor. This can go on for months and very often years before you are finally diagnosed with Interstitial Cystitis.

Interstitial Cystitis (IC) is typically described as a chronic inflammation of the bladder wall. Symptoms include, among other things, extreme urinary frequency, urgency, and pain. IC, once thought to be quite rare and occurring mostly in older women, is now frequently diagnosed in younger women, some men, and even some children. (Dogs and cats can also get IC.) There are varying degrees of IC (from mild to severe) and it can affect people of any age, race, or sex. However, IC is a disease that is most often diagnosed in women. (Although there is a current debate as to whether IC and Prostatitis are one and the same disease.) In 1987, it was estimated that approximately half a million people in the U.S. were suffering from IC. In 1997, just ten years later, the estimates are closer to two and a half million.

Unfortunately, IC is anything but a simple disease. No cause has been agreed upon. No treatment works for everyone. There is no known cure. It is very difficult to make blanket statements about IC, because there is little that has been proven scientifically. From diagnosis to treatments, controversy abounds. I don't have all the answers and certainly don't claim to. However, I have decided to share my experience and opinions regardless, with the hope that you will take from them what feels right to you and leave the rest behind.

As I sit here among my mounds of notebooks full of conversations among hundreds of IC patients and stacks of medical articles about IC, Prostatitis, and hospital-borne infections, I realize that I can put them all aside, at least for now, and simply write what I know; what I know to be true about this incurable and devastating disease "they" call Interstitial Cystitis. I choose for this book to be full of information that is not already "out there", that has not necessarily been "spoken", except maybe within the circles of IC patients themselves.

There is much mystery surrounding this disease. So little has been proven and not much can be said to be "known". There is risk in coming forward and saying what you know to be true, when not all the information has been proven scientifically or approved by the AMA as such. However, I take this risk freely, and beholden to no one (not the medical community, nor any organization or corporation) as many of my opinions are those held by many (but, of course, not all) IC patients. In fact, there will most likely be many IC patients who disagree with my opinions about what IC is and how to treat it. But that is okay. If, in your disagreement, you come to understand your IC better, then I am very pleased.

I write *To Wake In Tears* from a deep understanding of the suffering IC patients endure, not only from the disease itself, but also from the doctors, medical community, and others in their life as well. It is you, the IC patient, who I do not want to disappoint as I write this book. It is you who is important to me. It is you who I speak to now.

I share my story with you first because I know that there are many IC patients who have had similar experiences. It is worth telling if I can prevent at least one person from having to go through even a portion of what I (and so many others) have been through and/or at the very least let you know that you are not alone if you've already been through it yourself. It has been very difficult for me to write this part of the book. Mostly because of how upsetting it is to remember the physical pain, the emotional hurt, the anger, the stress, and the fear I've felt over the past three years. To remember...all the times...I woke in tears...

# Contents

Alternative ways....

Remember to breathe....

Finding your path...

"Believe nothing, no matter where you read it, or who said it, no matter if I have said it, unless it agrees with your own reason and your own common sense."
- Buddha

*The tears...*

# Chapter 1

$\blacklozenge$

# My Story

I've never been much of a crier. Fortunately for me, I never had much to cry about. I don't know if it was having three brothers that toughened me up or if it was just a fluke of nature, but when I was young and got hurt, I rarely cried. And until my father died when I was thirty, I never really had anything major to cry about emotionally either. Well...this was all about to change.

It was August of 1994 and the pain on my left side was becoming intolerable. I'd have to have the cyst removed. My gynecologist scheduled me for surgery the morning before she was to leave for her three week vacation. Neither one of us thought it should wait until she got back. After the surgery, I was told that, although she removed a number of small cysts, she was unable to understand why they were causing me so much pain. I was sent home that afternoon and my doctor left for her vacation. By that evening, I knew that something was terribly wrong.

Because I'd had an ovarian cyst when I was 23 with no complications and because this time I was physically unable to do the simple exercises described on the hospital discharge instructions, I knew enough to be concerned. In the days to follow I became more and more frightened knowing that the pain was not "normal" post-surgical pain. For the next two and a half weeks, I called my doctor's office every day and the emergency on-call physician every night. Since my file and the surgery report had not made it back to the doctor's office yet, and since my doctor was on vacation, it took a lot of phone calls and a couple of doctor visits to her associates in order to get someone to understand that something was seriously wrong. It turns out that the cyst originally causing the pain on my left side had ruptured, either during the surgery or immediately following. And so, two and a half weeks later, I was diagnosed with internal bleeding and peritonitis and taken immediately back into surgery. It was when I woke up from this second surgery that the nightmare really began. I remember waking up in recovery with the doctor and nurses by my side. My mom and my fiancée, Charlie, were in the room with us. They wanted to give me a shot for the pain and I was pleading with them "no...no...through the IV". I was already crying from the pain in my abdomen. The doctor told me that they were already giving me Demerol through the IV, but that I had to have this shot too or I would be in way too much pain. They rolled me over and gave me the shot as I squeezed Charlie's hand and screamed. They wanted me to stay in the hospital overnight, but of course, I wanted to go home. Charlie convinced me to stay by saying that he would stay with me. Okay, I said, I would stay. Before they took me up to my room, the doctor examined me one more time. I remember him telling me several times what a lucky girl I was. One more day, he was saying, over and over, shaking his head...and I wouldn't have made it.

I'll never forget that very first night. Clutching the metal bar attached to the wall next to the toilet with my left hand, the IV pole with my right, I sat most of the night, rocking back and forth in agony, trying to empty my bladder. I pulled the cord for the nurse. She explained that my bladder was irritated from the catheter, tired and beat up from the surgery. She tried to tell me not to worry. But I was worried. My bladder wouldn't work. I was terrified. It was September 17, 1994. The day I got IC.

Now at 31 years old, I had never even had a bladder infection before. And like most people, I had never even heard of Interstitial Cystitis. At this point, I had no idea what was wrong with me. I was sent home from the hospital the next day, only to be re-admitted two days later with a massive kidney/bladder infection. I was put on IV antibiotics for a couple of days and then sent home.

2

For the next several weeks, I went to see my new gynecologist complaining of bladder problems (extreme frequency, urgency, inability to empty bladder, inability to start the urine stream, blood in the urine) and pain in the pelvic/abdominal area since the surgery. He had my urine cultured and told me that they found all kinds of bacteria in the culture, some they could identify and some they could not. As I had already been on antibiotics after the surgery, he told me that he hoped it would clear up on it's own. I naively accepted this explanation without ever asking him WHY there was all this bacteria in my urine (as in WHERE did it come from, since it wasn't there before) or HOW it was going to clear up on it's own. But, I thought, I'd always been quite healthy and strong...maybe he was right. As the weeks went by, we both realized there was more to it than that and I was sent to a urologist for evaluation.

Now began the journey, or should I say the nightmare, of trying to get diagnosed. As most IC patients know, this is no easy task. I was sent to the head of urology at a prestigious hospital and was told that there was nothing wrong with my bladder. He told me I had emotional problems because my father had passed away the year before. I said, "I don't think so." He said that this happens to women, these "emotional problems", and it affects the bladder. This made no sense to me. But, I was new to this, so I tried to explain. "My bladder was normal prior to the surgery. Don't you think there might be a possibility that *maybe* something might have happened during the surgery, or as a result of the surgery, to cause these horrible symptoms I'm having?" I asked. "No", he said. "Okay...." I said. And I turned to leave his office. He stopped me at the door and insisted that "just in case" maybe I should let him examine me with an in-office cystoscopy. I tried to explain that with the two recent surgeries, I was in too much pain to try this procedure. He promised to be careful and assured me that this was the only way to find out if anything was really wrong. Of course I was desperate to get out of this pain and wanted to know what was wrong, so I agreed. This was a major mistake. *For most IC patients, an in-office cystoscopy is sheer torture.* I literally turned white, passed out, and got sick from the pain. It took me a couple weeks to get back to the pain level I was at prior to this cystoscopy.

This was my first experience with a urologist and this was my first misdiagnosis. On different occasions in the next several months I was told, by various doctors, that I had chronic pain syndrome, emotional problems causing my "bladder problems", a "spastic" bladder (that spontaneously decided to become "spastic"), and phantom pain from the shock of the peritonitis surgery. I was basically being told over and over again, in so many words, that this problem was in my head and that there was nothing they could do for me. Sadly, this is an extremely common experience for IC patients. Almost all of us, before being diagnosed, are told that we have nothing at all wrong with us or that the problem is "all in our heads". Many are referred to psychiatrists, instead of being treated as physically ill. It is a tragedy that still occurs to this day. I was somewhat fortunate to have such a dramatic onset to my IC. Whether the doctors believed me or not, I knew something was physically wrong, because my bladder was just fine before the surgery. So the search for an answer continued.

In the meantime, my quality of life was changing dramatically. Within the next six months my symptoms became worse and worse. Eventually I couldn't go to work at all because of the pain and the constant need to be in the bathroom. I lost my job about four months before getting diagnosed. During those four months I made numerous trips to the emergency room for the blood clots coming from my bladder. I was no longer "just" bleeding during urination. I had lost about twenty pounds and at 5'5" I weighed 94 pounds (my normal weight was 112-116). Anything I ate or drank caused severe pain, so I could barely do either. I was hunched over and could barely walk. I couldn't shower because the pain of the water hitting my body was more than I could bear. Nor could I sit in a bathtub. The pressure of even a couple inches of water would cause extreme pain. I had to sit, hunched over in tears, on a towel on the side of the tub and take a sponge bath. I averaged 75 trips to the bathroom a day. On bad days, my frequency was easily near 100. I couldn't lift a cup of water without causing severe pain. And through all this pain and bleeding, I was continually being told that there was nothing physically wrong with me.

At one point, after a desperate call to my gynecologist, he told me to meet him down at the hospital. Charlie drove me to the hospital as I cried in pain the entire way. We stopped four times on the way there (a half hour drive) so I could try to go to the bathroom. We finally got there and I was admitted. I was told that I couldn't have anything for the pain until they figured out exactly what was wrong with me. In walks the same urologist (the first one I'd seen) who had told me that there was nothing physically wrong with me and that I was having emotional problems causing my pain. I told my gynecologist that I didn't want that urologist to come near me, that he had physically hurt me the last time I saw him. He tells me that we have no choice, he was the only urologist available in the hospital that night, and that I had to be examined. So this urologist comes and sits down on the bed and presses his hand very firmly down onto my bladder and pushes in very hard. I screamed out loud in agony, and out of reflex, pushed his hand away. This was the first time in my entire life that I ever pushed a doctor's hand away from me. But the pain left me no choice. The urologist gets up off the bed and tells Charlie and my mom that I am refusing to be examined. He says that I have a problem getting along with doctors and that there is nothing at all wrong with my bladder. Of course I'm still hunched over in pain, crying on the bed. He tells them he thinks maybe I am anorexic because I am so thin. I try to tell him through the tears that part of the reason I am there at the hospital was because I was scared that I lost all this weight. And that if he knew anything about anorexia, he would realize that an anorexic would not be *trying* to gain weight or be worried that they were loosing weight. The gynecologist asks everyone to go out into the hallway to talk because he said I was getting too upset. Charlie is desperately trying to comfort me. I ask him to go out into the hall and find out what's going on. So now...the two resident doctors, my gynecologist, and this obnoxious urologist are out in the hall, right outside my hospital room, talking to my mom and my fiancée about me. I was furious at what had just happened and furious that they were all out there talking about me, instead of *to* me. I crawl out of the bed, still in tears from the pain this urologist had caused, push my IV pole and myself out into the hallway. My gynecologist saw me and tried to get me to get back into the bed. I refused and told him that they were all talking about me and that I wanted, and had a right, to hear what was going on. So they all come back into the room, just to get me to get back into the bed. My mom is still out in the hallway yelling at the urologist. She explained to him that she has known me my entire life and that if I said I was in pain, then I was in pain. She told him to prove to her that nothing was physically wrong with me and then, and only then, would she take me to see a psychiatrist. She said she would fly me around the world to see psychiatrists if he could prove to her that nothing was physically wrong with me. So when they all got back in the room, they agreed to set up a cat scan immediately.

I was taken downstairs with Charlie for the test. By the time we returned to the room, the gynecologist was there telling me that he wanted to open me up first thing in the morning. They noticed what they thought were some adhesions, a spot on my liver, and what looked like an inflamed ovary sitting on top of my bladder. He wanted to go in and check it out. Then he looks into my chart with the urologist and they ask me about blood in my urine from four years ago. I tell them I've never had blood in my urine in my life before this. They said "what about when you saw Dr. so and so". And I said "I've never even heard of this Dr. so and so. What are you talking about?!" We then realize that they had the wrong chart on me this whole time. There was another woman with my same name and they were using her chart. This is when I really got mad. I start screaming at them that they are using some other woman's chart. I look furiously at my gynecologist, as I start to get out of the hospital gown and into my clothes (in front of everyone mind you), and say "there's no f-in way I'm letting you guys touch me…you don't even know who I am!". He nodded his head silently as if he understood. One of the residents who was in the room said something about getting me discharged, as they all realized by now that I was leaving. The gynecologist waves him off, knowing that I had no intention of waiting until I got discharged to leave. My mom and Charlie are silent as they wheel me down the hallway to the elevator. I'm screaming and swearing at the doctors the whole way down the hall, down the elevator, and out to the car. Charlie takes me home. But I'm still in agony, I still don't know what is wrong with me, and I had no idea what to do next.

Within a week, we are back at the hospital. I felt I had no choice at the time. At least this gynecologist believed me before when I had internal bleeding and peritonitis, I thought, and he DID literally save my life. Prior to that awful night in the hospital, he had always been nice to me and at least he believed me when I said that I was in pain. It was the urologist that hurt me physically and had no idea what he was doing, I told myself. And it was the hospital's fault that they had the wrong chart on me, I decided. And my gynecologist DID have all my records and test results. These were all my rationalizations for going back one more time.

Once I was admitted and got to the room, a resident doctor wanted to examine me to see if I was bleeding vaginally or from the bladder. He used one of those metal instruments they use when you get a pap smear, but he didn't put any lubrication on it. I screamed out in pain when he tried to insert it and he got upset with me telling me that I *had* to let him examine me. I squeezed the nurses' hand and cried the whole time, but I let him examine me. When he was through, he told me that there was so much blood that he just couldn't tell. So it was all for nothing anyway. I asked for something for the pain and he said I had to wait until the nurse had time to get to me. I had to wait a couple more hours in the room before the nurse had time to hook me up to an IV. They still wouldn't give me anything for the pain.

When it was finally my turn to be hooked up to an IV for fluids, another horrible life threatening experience came out of nowhere. They turned the IV drip on too fast, telling me the whole time how I need to start drinking more because I was very dehydrated. And because I was very dehydrated, the IV drip was sending waves of cold up my arm. I kept telling them that it was too fast. They acted angry and annoyed with me and told me that if I would drink, I wouldn't be this dehydrated and that they had to get these fluids into me if I was to have surgery first thing in the morning. Within minutes of them leaving the room I started completely freaking out. My entire body was instantly covered in sweat, then I couldn't move my fingers, my hands got all cramped up and I started going "far away". I started screaming, "help!" and "I'm going to die!" and "please, please help me". Charlie was scared and didn't know what to do. He ran out into the hallway yelling for a nurse or doctor to come. Within seconds I was ripping off my hospital gown and I started rushing toward the bathroom. I heard voices behind me in the bathroom as I was violently throwing up. They were saying things like "is it green?", "yes, it's green". They called for a doctor and I heard them say I was having a seizure. I just kept throwing up while they put a sedative into my IV. And then finally…they turn down the IV drip (like I had asked them to do from the start). I crawled back into the bed and fell asleep.

The next morning we waited and waited for them to take me down to surgery. I was finally told that there was a mix up and that now I'm scheduled for later in the day. In the meantime, I got a call in the hospital room from the gynecologist who tells me that someone on the floor told him that I was smoking a cigarette in my hospital room. I say "WHAT?! WHY would I do that?!". I tell him a couple of times that, of course, I wasn't smoking in my hospital room and what was he talking about. He tells me about liability and how I ruined his whole Saturday (because I guess he would have been off that day). So I told him that he could leave then, because there was no way I was going to let him touch me now. I left the hospital that day...that hospital where I got IC from in the first place, and never went back.

Within the next week I decide to try the next best hospital in the city. I naively have my records transferred, thinking that this will help my new doctor figure out what's wrong with me. I wanted them to know what I had been through with the two surgeries, because I still felt that the second surgery had something to do with what was wrong with me. I

8

had no idea at this point that there was absolutely no record of my second surgery in my file. And as it turned out, unbeknownst to me, the new gynecologist I went to see was a friend of my old gynecologist.

I was instantly treated like I was crazy, again, at this new hospital, though I didn't know why at the time. The new gynecologist considered the possibility of adhesions, yet told me I had chronic pain syndrome and wanted me to "get some help". He did say he was "willing" to do an exploratory laporoscopy, but I refused, knowing that he didn't believe me and thought I was nuts.

In the meantime, that same week, I had yet another trip to the emergency room for the pain and blood coming from my bladder. This time they lost my sample and then put my chart in the wrong basket, so I had to wait four hours before seeing a doctor. When he finally came in, he directed the entire conversation to Charlie, because, of course, he thought I was some hysterical female (judging from what he must have been reading in my chart). He tells Charlie a bunch of stuff about chronic pain syndrome and how they aren't sure the blood is really coming from my bladder. (As if at 31 years old I couldn't tell the difference between my period and my bladder bleeding! Geesh!) I asked him for something for the pain. After all, I had been lying on this hard, uncomfortable hospital gurney for the past four hours, in pain the entire time, and I kept having to walk down a big, long hallway to the bathroom every five to ten minutes. The urologist tells me "we don't just hand out pain medication to anyone who asks" and again suggests the chronic pain clinic. I "jump" down off the hospital cart (well…okay…I kind of slid) and explain to him that I graduated Magna Cum Laude with a master's degree from Case Western Reserve University. Not only am I a licensed counselor myself, I tell him, I am NOT stupid. I tell him that I KNOW what he's trying to say to me. He finally looks at me and admits that I probably know more about Chronic Pain Syndrome than he does and suggests that we do a cystoscopy under anesthesia to find out what's really going on. Finally! This was the first time the guy even looked at me the whole time he was in the room with us. And the first time he even considered the possibility that there may be a physical cause to my pain.

Even after this experience, I still decided (if you can believe it), to let the head of urology at this hospital do a cystoscopy under anesthesia and examine my bladder. I needed to know what was wrong with me. The morning I went in for this cystoscopy, the head of urology had some emergency to take care of, so at the last minute they decided to have one of the resident urologists do my cystoscopy. We didn't find this out until literally minutes before they took me in to surgery. What I am about to write sends shivers up my spine. It has taken me weeks to get up the courage to remember and think about this enough to write about it. When I woke up from this cystoscopy was the worst experience and the worst pain that I've ever been through in my entire life. I still have nightmares about it three years later. It was worse than the pain from the in-office cystoscopy where I turned white, passed out, and got sick. The resident urologist had decided to leave the catheter in after surgery, so from the very second I became conscious in the recovery room, I was in sheer agony. There I was with a raw, bleeding bladder with a catheter sucking urine out it. The pain was excruciating and I felt the most urgent need to go the bathroom. I screamed and cried to the nurse in the recovery room. She gave me another bag of Demerol through my IV and told me that the doctor wanted the catheter to stay in. I kept screaming and crying REALLY loud, to where Charlie heard me all the way down the hall. Charlie, of course, came running into the recovery room and the nurse, believe it or not, was grateful to see him, thinking that he could calm me down. The pain was too much. I couldn't help screaming. The nurse gave me another bag of Demerol through the IV and tried to reach the resident urologist. (Throughout this time, I felt no effects from the Demerol whatsoever because the pain was so intense. I remember hearing the nurse tell Charlie that she had already given me three bags and that she just couldn't give me anymore.) The resident urologist was in surgery and couldn't come to the phone. So they decided to wheel me up to the chronic pain floor to get me out of the recovery room. I guess I was scaring the other patients. The nurse was beside herself and seemed quite upset with my constant screaming and crying. But there was nothing I could do. What did she think...that I wanted to make a complete spectacle of myself? Charlie was trying to keep me calm. He was telling me...."just listen to my voice and hang on" and he was singing to me, real soft, the songs that he had written for me.

As they wheeled me up to the 8th floor with this catheter still in me causing excruciating pain...over the bumps in the hallways and the bumps in the elevator, we pass by my mom in the hallway. It was heart-wrenching to see her face as she saw me on the cart in agony. I yelled to Charlie to get her away and that I didn't want her to see me like this. I thought I was going to die just from the pain alone. I was crying as hard as I have ever cried, begging them to take out the catheter and let me try to go to the bathroom myself. Finally, over two hours later upstairs in the room, the nurse came in and removed the catheter. I immediately went in and sat on the toilet for another hour just rocking back and forth in pain, leaned over with my head on Charlie's lap, until the resident urologist came up to the room and called me out of the bathroom "to talk". He barely apologizes and explains that he thought the catheter would help me. And how lucky I am because so many women have it worse than I did. He gave me some anti-spasmodic medication and sent me home. I never took them. Mostly because I STILL had no idea what was wrong with me.

I requested a copy of my medical records and that was when we discovered that there was no record at all of my second surgery. Oh...I had the bills for it and the insurance receipts saying that the hospital had been paid for the surgery, but there was no surgical report. No record at all that I had ever had internal bleeding, peritonitis, or a ruptured cyst. No record of any of the medications I had been given. No record of my physical complaints or the doctor's comments about them. I guess the liability issue of the first doctor missing the cyst that ruptured and the fact that I came so close to dying caused the second doctor (in the same practice) to "forget" to write all of this down. I called the records department of the hospital and spoke to a very nice, well-meaning woman. She checked and double-checked and then confirmed to me that there was no record that I had even been in the hospital that day and certainly no surgical report on file. She was as shocked as I was. Of course this is against the law in Ohio, but obviously that made no difference. Several months later I asked an attorney to look into this situation and miraculously a one page surgical report appeared at the attorney's office. It was completely illegible, only partially filled out, and basically said nothing except that I had had a laporoscopy. The names of the people present in the operating room that day were completely illegible. The report also was not dated or signed. The attorney said we had no case because we couldn't prove anything. It is interesting to note that the attorney received different medical records than I did when I requested them as a patient. And I learned another lesson as well. Prior to this experience, it had never occurred to me to pay attention to whether a doctor was writing down the truth of what was happening in my file or whether he was keeping track of the medications that he prescribed or anything of the sort.

Out of desperation, I went out of state to a uro-gynecologist for yet another laporoscopy and cystoscopy. It had been about six weeks since my last cystoscopy. It had taken us that long to find a doctor and come up with a plan. I actually made the long car ride to the airport, the walk through the airport, a flight to Chicago, and a drive to the hotel near the hospital in this miserable condition. The traveling was agony (as any IC patient understands) and the amount of bathroom stops was phenomenal, but I was determined (or should I say desperate) to find out what was wrong with me. When we finally made it out there and met the doctor in person, he started talking to me like I'm a crazy person. He asked Charlie to wait out in the hall while he asks me some questions. He asks me all kinds of personal (and mostly emotional-type) questions and then tells me that he thinks I have a very low tolerance for pain because he could barely examine me. I look him right in the eye and tell him, "I'm sorry, but you are so wrong. I actually have a very high tolerance for pain. And how would you know anyway since you just met me?" I'm highly annoyed with him at this point and very disappointed, to say the least. Then we met in his office with Charlie and he admitted to us that he spoke with his "friend" back in Cleveland about my case. His friend was the head of urology at the last hospital, the one that I never even met because he ended up having an emergency that morning. I tell him that I never actually met this guy he spoke to about me. And we both start desperately explaining to him what had happened in Cleveland and about the missing surgical report. Okay, he says, he's willing to do the cystoscopy and laporoscopy to find out what's going on. We left his office and I was in tears. My messed up chart had made it to Chicago and now this guy thinks I'm crazy too! And after all the pain I had been through to get there. I just couldn't return home without knowing what was wrong with me. We went ahead and let him do the surgery. This time the diagnosis was Severe Interstitial Cystitis. I was given a prescription for a tricyclic anti-depressant, pyridium, and pain medication (enough for about a week) and was sent home, or should I say, back to the hotel. As I sat there rocking back and forth in pain on the hotel bed, trying to get comfortable, leaning forward on a mound of pillows we had them bring up to the room, clueless from the Demerol and anesthesia...Charlie told me what the doctor had told him. The doctor never spoke to me after the surgery. I never saw him again. I think maybe he felt bad that he had treated me like a "nut" when we first got out there. I don't think he wanted to face me after he saw the inside of my bladder. In any case, I listened to what the doctor had told Charlie. He described the inside of my bladder as looking like Korea after the war. (Generally, when diagnosing IC, they have to distend the bladder to examine the lining for pinpoint hemorrhages. For me, I had bleeding upon initial instillation of even a small amount of liquid. My bladder lining was raw, "sparing no area" according to the surgical report.) I listened to all of this and yet still knew nothing at all about what was wrong with me or how to deal with it. Why was my bladder raw? Why was I in so much pain? And what about all these other symptoms....what did THEY have to do with my bladder? Would I get well? Could I get well? I didn't understand. All I knew was I wanted to go home. All I cared about at the time was that I had two more car rides, a plane ride, many trips to the bathroom and a lot of pain before I was back in my own bed again. This was all I could think about at the time. It didn't register yet that I had just been told I had an incurable bladder disease.

I was referred by the doctor in Chicago to a local urologist for a follow-up appointment, but could not get in for another six weeks. So here I was...no pain medication left and at least five more weeks to go until I could get in to see the urologist. And so began my quest for understanding Interstitial Cystitis.

One of the first things I did was get on the computer and do a search on Interstitial Cystitis. I found an on-line support group for IC and printed out dozens of articles off the web. By the time I went to my follow-up appointment, I had read Dr. Gillespie's "You Don't Have to Live With Cystitis", Drs. Whitmore and Chalker's "Overcoming Bladder Disorders", many medical articles on IC, and had "spoken" with many IC patients via the computer. I was by no means an "expert", but I was no longer completely ignorant about IC either.

After surviving the next five weeks with no pain medication, the urologist wanted me to try bladder instillations as a first line of treatment. (Bladder instillations are when they instill medications directly into the bladder via catheter.) He claimed that this helped most of his patients and that this was his first line of treatment. I explained to him that I had spoken with several IC patients that were not helped by bladder instillations. And that actually, many of them told me they made their symptoms worse. I was not ready to try any invasive procedures I told him, especially with the risk of making my bladder worse. "Could we not look at some of the alternatives?" I naively asked. He said that I must not have been in enough pain or I would try the instillations. So "no instillations, no pain medication" is exactly what he told me. I left his office and have not been to a urologist since.

I had no idea what to do next. Once you finally get diagnosed, there is this strange mix of emotion. You are, all at once, relieved (to know what it is), justified (your sanity has been confirmed), terrified (that you have an incurable disease), confused (now what do you do?), angry, and alone. To top it all off, many IC patients, at the time of diagnosis, as well as after, experience a great lack of concern, compassion, sympathy, and understanding from others. I was no exception. After my diagnosis, there were no phone calls, no visits, no cards or flowers, no apologies for all the doubt and disbelief. I know that many of us have lost "friends", spouses or significant others, and family members, due to our experience with IC. Please don't think you are alone in this experience. The lack of understanding of this disease causes so many problems for IC patients to deal with aside from their physical pain.

Aside from dealing with other people in our lives who don't understand, the fact that doctors have very little understanding of IC is, of course, a major problem. Sadly, there are still many doctors out there who don't even believe that IC exists. Up until about twenty years ago, IC was still considered a disease caused by the neurosis of women (even though 10% of the sufferers were, and are, men). Somehow women were, by the sheer power of their minds and emotions, mysteriously causing their bladders to bleed. Tragically, some doctors today still believe this. Even the doctors who do recognize IC as a disease, admittedly don't understand the cause nor can they offer a cure. So what do we do?

Well...living with the pain is definitely not an option. Living with the constant need to be in the bathroom is also not an option. From the moment I was diagnosed, I refused to believe that I was going to have IC for the rest of my life. I was determined to understand IC, get rid of it, and get my life back. I've spent the last three years doing just that. This book is a compilation of what I have learned from talking to hundreds and hundreds of other IC patients daily over the past three years as a co-leader of an on-line IC support group, studying the IC research, working with medical intuitive/psychic healers, and my own personal experience of having Severe IC...and recovering.

# Chapter 2

———◆———

# I Remember

"It is such a secret place, the land of tears."
- Antoine de Saint Exupery
*The Little Prince*

With an ever-present urgency and constant burning pain, sleep was a luxury found only through exhaustion. I was almost afraid to fall asleep for the pain that awaited me when I awoke. The first words to cross my lips every morning were "everything hurts, everything hurts!". Over and over I would repeat it, as if I had no control. The pain just seemed to force the words through my breath. With tears in my eyes, I would crawl out of bed to the bathroom. Another pain-filled day alone in the bathroom lie ahead. Another day of searching for a doctor who treats IC and/or someone who would prescribe something for the pain. Another day filled with worry, searching for some answers and for some relief.

You would think that after finally getting diagnosed, especially with a severe case of IC, that I could finally find some relief from the pain. But this was still very difficult to do. I still had to find a doctor in my area who understood IC enough to know that it can be extremely painful. The urologist who was supposedly the "IC expert" here did not believe in prescribing pain medication to IC patients. (Which shows you what an expert he was!) I called the ICA (Interstitial Cystitis Association), but they didn't know any urologists in my area that they could recommend.

I called every urologist in the phone book (except for the two idiots I had already seen) and asked if they treated IC patients. No luck. I called every pain clinic in the city and asked if they treated IC pain. Still no luck. They had never even heard of IC. (I know you're shocked.) Finally, through a friend of Charlie's, I found a compassionate internist who understood that having a raw bladder was painful enough to warrant pain medication.

By the way, it is quite common to feel uncomfortable asking for pain medication. I know many IC patients, who, like myself, were afraid to ask after getting turned down by several doctors who didn't believe they were in pain. We are often made to feel like we are crazy or treated like we're drug addicts or something. We are humiliated. It then becomes more difficult to ask. But you have to ask. You have to find someone who is willing to listen and get you out of pain. I remember Charlie and I talking about how we would do anything, pay any amount of money, just to get me out of pain. And at the same time, I also remember never wanting to take the pain medication once I finally had some. I was afraid of feeling worse in other ways from the side effects (the nausea, the stomach pain, the dizziness). And it rarely took away all the pain anyway. So then I would have both the side effects AND the bladder symptoms and pain. I was always afraid to take pain medication when I was alone because of the overdose-type allergic reactions I had right after getting IC. There was also the fact that I was afraid of running out and not being able to get anymore. I remember talking with other IC patients about how we all kept an emergency supply of pain medication for those days that the pain was well past 10 on a 1-10 scale.

The first couple months after getting diagnosed were filled with fear. I remember so much fear...and so many tears. I remember the swelling in my abdomen and bladder being so severe that I couldn't stand up straight. I was always hunched over, barely able to walk. I was extremely thin and looked deathly ill. Well...deathly ill and three months pregnant. (You know the look.) I remember not being able to lift a glass of water from the pain it caused my bladder. The remote control for the television was way too heavy to have sitting on my belly, or even on my leg for that matter. If someone walked across the floor I could feel the vibration in my bladder. I remember screaming out in pain if someone brushed up against the bed. Any type of movement caused pain.

Riding in a car was a torturous experience that I tried to avoid as much as possible. The urgency was extreme because of the irritation from the constant vibrations. The vibration and bumps along the road can cause excruciating pain. I remember talking with other IC patients about our fear of traffic jams. (See...you're not the only one.) I was always afraid to go in the car with someone other than Charlie driving. Someone who may not have understood that I needed to stop constantly, and very often, immediately. I made the mistake of going in a car with someone other than Charlie driving only once.

There were a lot of new fears to deal with. The fear of not being able to make it to the next bathroom was just one of them. There was the fear of not being able to "go", and then the fear of the burning pain while I WAS "going", and then there were the bladder spasms (or sharp, shooting pains) immediately AFTER "going". I remember the relentless, burning pain in my bladder. The stabbing, sharp pain that made me afraid to move or breathe for fear of causing more. I remember feeling really alone in that pain. I remember feeling that no one understood how terrible it was.

I remember a lot of waiting. Waiting for doctors to return my call. Waiting for prescriptions to be called in or waiting for them to be filled. Waiting for culture results. Waiting in waiting rooms. Waiting for pain medication to work. Waiting to feel better. Waiting to fall asleep. Waiting to pee. Waiting for spasms to stop. Waiting for a cure. Oh yeah...I definitely remember a lot of waiting.

I remember waiting for Charlie to get home from work to get me something to drink. I remember not being able to lift anything to get it

19

for myself. There were even times that opening the refrigerator was too difficult. I remember having to eat on plastic dishes and drink from plastic cups. Every morning Charlie would fill several plastic cups with distilled water and put them on the top shelf of the refrigerator, where it was easier for me to lift them up.

I remember being awake in the bathroom at 2:00am. Sitting there with nothing coming out. Scared and in pain. Extremely frustrated and exhausted. Feeling like I was the only person in the entire world who was awake. I remember not being able to get comfortable enough to go to sleep. The constant urgency had me always returning to the bathroom. And getting the rest of my body comfortable was no picnic either. I remember not being able to sleep on my left side. Not only would it cause pain in my bladder and abdomen, it would cause tremendous pain in my hip and leg as well.

I remember my nightstand being covered with prescription bottles and how the television was on twenty-four hours a day. I remember how I would sit there with the volume so low that you could barely hear it. I didn't feel well enough to actually watch. But it was company during the day when Charlie was at work and at night when he was asleep.

I remember spending a lot of time watching Charlie sleep. I was so envious. I found it hard not to be upset that he couldn't "be" with me during all those long, lonely hours in the middle of the night. I couldn't help wishing that he could hold my hand through all the pain, even though I knew it was impossible. After all, he did have to go to work and he WAS totally taking care of me. From the grocery shopping and the errands, to all the cooking, cleaning, and laundry, Charlie did absolutely *everything* for me. And without a single complaint...ever. Yet I still couldn't help feeling upset when he was unable to be there for me. That's how much pain I was in...I was just NOT myself.

I remember not feeling like myself in so many ways. Being in pain all the time with very little sleep was certainly no help. While I was sick I was....I don't know....different. I was much more nervous about things that normally would not have made me nervous. I was bothered by things that normally wouldn't have bothered me. It was as if I had lost my strength, my inner peace...my self. I just didn't feel like myself. I remember I didn't like how I felt.

I remember the glands under my arms being so swollen that I could see them in the mirror. I could barely lift either arm and putting on deodorant just wasn't an option. (Pleasant huh?) I remember Charlie washing my hair in the sink because I couldn't lift my arms high enough to wash it myself. I remember how nauseous I felt with my head in the sink. The glands at the top of both my legs were also very swollen and clearly visible. It was painful to walk or even have my underwear pressing against them. I used to get so upset sitting on the bed because I kept sliding forward and then my underwear would pull and press at my swollen glands. This is just one of those stupid, irritating, yet painful, things I remember about when I was really sick with IC. I remember constantly adjusting the mounds of pillows we had on the bed. I was forever trying to get comfortable.

I remember that every time I ate anything, the pressure of the food in my stomach, pressing further on...well...everything, caused so much pain that I was afraid to eat. The more I ate, the more pressure and pain. I remember not wanting to drink much of anything either because any amount of urine in my bladder was like a five alarm fire. I remember feeling really nauseous a lot, especially when my bladder was full.

I remember how the pain and urgency absorbed all my attention. I rarely spoke to anyone besides Charlie, but when I did, I remember how difficult it was to concentrate on what they were saying. It was difficult to care about what they were talking about. All I cared about, all I could care about, was the unrelenting pain, pressure, and urgency.

I remember the "poison pains". That's what Charlie and I used to call them. Those sharp, shooting, burning pains through the intestines that take your breath away. The ones that make you feel like you ate acid the day before. When, in an instant, your body is covered with sweat and you "go far away" like when you're about to pass out. Afraid to move or take a breath...sitting there doubled over on the toilet...afraid of, well, dying, quite frankly. And this is what they call Irritable Bowel?! This was much worse than something I would call "irritable". This was extremely painful and very scary every time it happened. For me, this was part of the daily torture of having IC. And not knowing when it was going to happen was all just part of the fun. I remember Charlie rushing to get me a glass of water and a cool washcloth to put on the back of my neck to "bring me back". I remember all those times I was by myself and Charlie was at work; how completely frightening it was...and how painful. I would pray and pray and pray. I would call Charlie on the portable phone and he would talk me through it. I remember being completely exhausted afterwards.

I remember Charlie sitting with me in the bathroom, on the floor or on the counter...playing his guitar and singing to me. Trying to help me relax and to not be so afraid. Keeping me company. Trying to get my mind off the pain. Not knowing what to do any more than I did. But he was there. He stuck by me every step of the way. Believing in me...supporting me...loving me...marrying me even! Even in the midst of my IC. Not knowing for sure if I would ever get better, Charlie married me just the same. I remember how that surprised certain people.

I remember looking for a doctor, but being afraid to go to one. Afraid of what they were going to do to me. Afraid they were going to hurt me more. Afraid of them treating me like I was nuts. And at the same time, afraid of them telling me something else was wrong with me. But mostly I was afraid of them touching me at all, causing even more pain, that would take days to recover from.

I remember how we used to joke. Because I lived, for the better part of three years, on my bed or in the bathroom, we used to joke about how

I was a bubble-child (like in the old John Travolta movie *The Boy In The Plastic Bubble*). Though it really wasn't very funny that I was rarely well enough to leave the house. We used to joke that my best friend was the maintenance man at our apartment complex, because I saw him more than I saw anyone else (except for Charlie of course). But it really wasn't very funny how many "friends" I lost for having IC.

We also used to joke about my other "best friend"...the heating pad. We actually named it "the wooby" from the movie *Mr. Mom*. (Do you think we watch too much television?) For at least a year and a half, my heating pad was on all day and all night. It was always there, faithfully waiting for me, when I got back to the bed. We joked a lot about my constant companion, but it really wasn't very funny that I was in even more pain when I didn't have it on.

We used to joke about my blue pants and how I wore them everyday. (You know that one pair of pants? The ones that are stretched out with no elastic left at the waist. The ones that don't put any pressure on your swollen belly. I know you have a pair too.) Well...my blue pants were these old pajama bottoms from Victoria's Secret that looked like leggings. There was no elastic on the waist and a small amount of spandex throughout kept them from falling to the floor. The only time I didn't have them on during the day was when they were in the washing machine. We joked a lot about those blue pants, but it really wasn't very funny that I had a closet full of beautiful clothes that I could no longer wear.

We used to joke about how I could never remember that I had seen certain movies because I was on pain medication when we watched them. But it really wasn't very funny that we wasted all that money on video rentals. (Just kidding! That's not why it wasn't funny.)

We used to joke that I actually lived in the bathroom and how maybe we should put a television in there for me. But it really wasn't very funny that I made over 100 trips to the bathroom on a bad day. We used to joke about my pillow mountain on the bed and how I would constantly re-arrange them. But it wasn't very funny how I had to struggle all the time to find some semblance of comfort. We used to joke about so many things while I was so sick. Because, as they say…sometimes you have to laugh…so you don't cry.

As I sit here writing this, I keep picturing myself alone in the bathroom, bleeding, in pain, not knowing what to do, not knowing if I would ever get better. What would I want to read? What would I want to hear? I wanted some answers. I wanted to be out of pain. I wanted to know that there was a way to get well. I wanted some understanding of this disease so that I could fight back. So that I could get "me" back. Some type of treatment that would help cure me of this awful disease. I also wanted to know that people cared. I wanted to know that they understood…at least a little bit…of what I was going through. I wished that they could feel the pain, just for a minute, so that they could know how bad it really was. (I think one of the toughest things about IC is getting people to understand the pain.) I wanted to know that I wasn't alone. I wanted to be out of pain. I wanted my bladder to work again. I wanted my life back!

*Understanding begins...*

# Chapter 3

---◆---

## Searching For Answers

Now…how I came to my understanding of IC has more to do with desperation than anything else. When you're in severe pain every minute of every day, the kind of pain that pain medications barely touch, when you can't urinate and your bladder is bleeding huge blood clots…I'm sorry…you are desperate. There is just no way around it. This desperation I felt to get well, the severity of the physical pain, the tremendous fear I had that no one could (or would) help me get well…all led me down an uncharted path.

Since I had always been rather healthy, I had no reasons, prior to getting IC, to doubt the medical community. It wasn't that I thought that doctors were "gods" or anything, but I did have some trust that they knew what they were doing. I guess it was something that I had just never given much thought. When I got hurt playing softball, for example, and was taken to the emergency room, I wasn't scared that they didn't know what they were doing or that they were going to hurt me physically more so than I already was. This just wasn't in my thinking. I believed that if you had an infection, you took an antibiotic. That if you went to the doctor because you didn't know what was wrong with you, that he/she would be able to tell you what it was and then give you something to help. I considered them "the experts". Alternative medicine, vitamins and herbs…they were all well and good, I had thought, but they were for minor physical ailments or for health maintenance or prevention, not for "serious" illness. This is just what I had always thought. I was like most people of my generation who were taught to believe in, listen to, and "check with your" doctor. We are told this every day on countless television commercials, on the news, in magazines, and on the radio.

So what do you do when your doctors have no answers? When they tell you there is no cure? When the treatments they offer are painful and invasive and only offer the possibility of short-term relief? What do you do after being mistreated and misdiagnosed by numerous doctors? When they've hurt you physically and then tell you it's in your head? What do you do when your doctor says stupid things like "IC is one of those diseases where we don't understand the cause nor do we have the cure, but we do know how to treat it"? What do you do when you realize that your doctor is just "practicing" on you?

Well...this is where I was coming from, desperate and in pain...with a very recent loss of faith in a medical community that had no real answers for me. Whether they had put me through previous torture or not, whether I was angry and hated them at the time or not...the fact still remained that they offered no cure. So I looked for answers elsewhere. I decided that I would figure this out myself. I first looked to my new IC friends on line and learned how they got IC, what treatments they had tried and what treatments had worked for them. *Some of the most valuable information I've learned about IC has come from other IC patients.*

One of the first things I learned from talking to other IC patients was that I was definitely not alone in how I got IC. My very first day on line I immediately found others who had the same experience. There are hundreds, probably thousands of other women who got IC immediately following surgery. This is rarely, if ever, discussed by physicians nor is it mentioned in the IC literature. (Shocked again...eh?) The reason for this is conjecture of course. However, I do have some ideas. I know that the liability issue is a definite possibility and ignorance is definitely another. And though I'm quite sure that physicians do not want to alarm their patients unnecessarily, it does concern me that every day women are having surgery and are not being told about IC as a possible risk. It is also a shame that the IC patient has no recourse with the law against the hospital (i.e., the liability issue). They are left damaged by the surgery with no way to prove it legally because the cause of IC has yet to be "proven".

28

Many IC patients, like myself, had some type of "female" surgery (e.g., hysterectomy, ovarian cysts, fibroids, tubal ligations, endometriosis) immediately prior to getting IC. Though some IC patients have a dramatic onset immediately following other types of surgery, and dental surgery, as well. It seems that the other most common way people get IC is following repeated urinary tract infections. (Or sometimes even one big UTI can trigger the onset of IC.) Eventually, one day, the patient will have symptoms where no infection is found in routine cultures and they will be told they have IC. (This is because IC has often been considered to be "non-bacterial cystitis".) In my observations, these are the two most common ways people get IC...though there most certainly are other ways. For example, recently I am hearing of younger woman who noticed their IC symptoms began following their first sexual experience. Some IC patients have no idea how they got IC, they just woke up one day in pain and have had IC ever since. Or maybe they have some guesses as to how they got sick, but they aren't quite sure. But, if asked, I have learned, that many IC patients can tell you how they got IC. Most often, they're not asked.

Another thing I learned quickly after talking to other IC patients is that we are all so different. Not only do we vary with regard to symptoms, we also vary with regard to which treatments work and which don't. It is really in this mystery that we are alone. That nobody has the answers. This disease manifests itself in very individual ways. What is an answer for one person may not be the answer for you. We are truly alone in this sense, and therefore we must look to ourselves for the answers. I realized that I could learn a lot from others, but I still had to find my own way.

# Chapter 4

———————◆———————

# What is IC? & Why is it all so confusing?

There are many factors contributing to the confusion about IC. First and foremost is that there is still no clear definition of IC. The definition of IC that exists today (1998) remains the same as the diagnostic criteria used in a study by the National Institute of Health. They devised a list of diagnostic criteria in order to collect data on this mysterious bladder disease. Hence, the "official" diagnostic criteria does not necessarily include every person who has IC. You don't necessarily have to fit each one of the criteria to have IC. Therefore, just because your urologist looked inside your bladder through cystoscopy and told you that you don't have IC, it does not necessarily mean that you don't have IC. I know IC patients who had several cystoscopies before they were officially diagnosed. Their urologist did not see the "hallmark" signs of IC, and therefore did not diagnose IC, even though all of their other symptoms may have pointed to IC. So the patients remained undiagnosed until their IC progressed enough for their urologist to see the cracks and pinpoint bleeding in their bladder lining upon distention.

At the same time, there is an argument that says IC is both over-diagnosed and under-diagnosed. Under-diagnosed by closed-minded doctors who still don't admit that there is a physical cause to this dreadful disease. And over-diagnosed by those doctors trying to give a "name" to a suffering patient without necessarily covering all the bases in terms of excluding other diagnoses. The reason for this is that IC still remains a diagnosis of exclusion. Typically, all other illness is ruled out, and then and only then, can IC be "truly" diagnosed.

With no clear definition of the disease itself, there is also, of course, no clear definition of what it means to be "cured" of IC either. How long do you have to be "well" before you are considered cured of IC? I know many IC patients who have had long periods (e.g., 2-5 years) of remission and then their IC comes back. What if a person's bladder symptoms are gone, but they still have other "related" problems. Should we consider them "cured"? What if they are "cured" as long as they remain on certain medications? Does this count?

One urologist at an IC support group meeting was asked the following. "With the treatment approaches you are using, what would you say your success rate is in your patients achieving remission?" His answer, I fear, would be typical. He believed his treatment approaches (of bladder instillations and various medications) were fairly successful in helping his IC patients into remission. "By what criteria are you measuring "remission"?", he was asked. He said, "Well...I assume they're in remission because they never come back." This had me laughing out loud. These poor urologists have no idea the reasons we don't go back! (Doctors rarely, if ever, call their patients to find out why they don't come back. This is not unique among urologists of course, this applies to most doctors. They don't have the time to follow up with patients. Most doctors barely have ten minutes to spend with you in the examining room, let alone call you on the phone to find out why you haven't come back in to see them.)

Another confusing factor is that we are all at different points with our IC in terms of diagnosis, symptoms, and treatment. Some are recently diagnosed, while others have had IC for years. (Actually, some who are recently diagnosed may have had IC for years because of the length of time it usually takes to get diagnosed.) Some IC patients have gone through treatments that made their bladders worse and maybe they are now having a tougher time trying to heal. Some have been in and out of remission, but now the treatment they're using is no longer helping. Some had a dramatic onset, while others seem to develop IC more gradually. There are some IC patients who have many IC-related symptoms that came immediately with their IC, while other IC patients develop these IC-related symptoms over time. Some IC patients experience both. They get many IC-related symptoms right away, and then develop new ones over time.

As previously mentioned, IC-related symptoms also vary among individual IC patients. While some IC patients may be dealing with severe fibromyalgia symptoms, others may be experiencing kidney stones or kidney infections. Some may be dealing with TMJ and mouth problems, where other IC patients have IBS and Chronic Fatigue Syndrome. Specific bladder symptoms like frequency, urgency, and pain, for example, can range in intensity from non-existent (or mild) to severe.

More confusion is caused by the fact that some IC patients experience flares and remissions and others, like myself, seem to get IC and then just have it (without experiencing flares and remissions). Very often this is not mentioned in the IC literature. There are those of us out here who don't experience what others call "flares". We just have symptoms all the time that are basically the same all the time. Some days might be a little bit better than others, but that's about it. So when "they" describe IC symptoms as those that "wax and wane", it is very confusing to those of us who don't have that experience.

Some IC patients experience catching every little cold and flu bug that is going around, while others believe that their immune system is working overtime and they therefore get "normal" illnesses (e.g., colds and flu) less often. Some experience remission during pregnancy, some do not, and others get worse. Some IC patients stay in remission after they deliver, others do not. You get the idea.

As I mentioned before, the fact that no treatment works for everyone also causes confusion. We all respond differently to different treatments. When it comes to IC treatments, research control groups are very often not possible which makes it difficult to determine the effectiveness of a treatment. This is because IC treatments are typically invasive and painful. Bladder instillations using DMSO is a perfect example of this because not only is it invasive and very often painful, it also causes the patient to smell like garlic for 2-3 days afterward. Therefore, it would be difficult to have a control group to study the effectiveness of DMSO.

Also, IC research groups are probably not uniform to begin with, since the definition and diagnosis of IC is still not uniform. So, in my opinion, the research results we have thus far may not be all that accurate. Regardless of the accuracy of the research results, *much of the research is still looking at tiny pieces of the puzzle where IC is concerned.* Western medicine often looks at disease in small parts, forgetting that the whole body functions together as a unit. But this is only part of the problem. There are so many reasons for the confusion when it comes to the etiology of IC.

When you read the medical research, you will find many different theories about IC. There are theories that say IC is caused by a defect in the protective glycosaminoglycan (GAG) layer or the bladder lining. There are theories that say IC is an auto-immune disease, a connective tissue disease, or an allergic reaction. Some theories recognize the activation of mast cells in the bladders of IC patients. Some say that hormones are involved, while others believe that IC is caused by a previous bacterial infection. There are still others who believe that IC is due to nerve dysfunction and/or a previous back injury. There is also research looking into a toxic substance in the urine of IC patients or a malfunction of the kidneys producing something toxic to the bladder. Some say that IC is a result of many different disease processes. There is research in all kinds of areas trying to determine the etiology, or cause, of IC. I'm sure many of you have read the medical articles that all seem to have conflicting results. I hardly consider myself qualified to review the medical literature in any in-depth manner, and therefore will not attempt to do so here. I leave it up to you to read the research articles and draw your own conclusions, which is as it should be.

Even after reading all the literature, we, as individuals, still have to determine what WE think IC is, how we got it, and how we can get rid of it. The research results remain unclear as of this writing. And, in my opinion, until the medical community provides us with a clear description of what IC is, we are basically on our own. Until "they" provide us with a "scientifically proven" cause and/or cure for IC, we have to rely on, or operate based on, what we believe IC to be. Obviously, this can be tricky even after you read all the medical literature available on IC.

One thing I can tell you is that many of these medical articles have in common their description of IC. Most all of them, until very recently, describe only bladder symptoms, such as bladder and pelvic pain, urinary urgency and frequency. But IC is so much more than simply cystitis-like symptoms. To say that IC is "a chronic inflammation of the bladder wall", as it is so often put, is putting it very mildly. *And herein lies a major point of this book, as well as, in my opinion, one of the major downfalls of much of the IC research, and therefore, treatment. IC is not just a bladder disease.*

# Chapter 5

------------------- ◆ -------------------

# Other Symptoms of IC

A major confusing factor in my search for a diagnosis was the fact that I had numerous other symptoms aside from the bladder symptoms. And even after I was diagnosed, I still didn't know what to make of all these other symptoms. I read the IC research and saw no mention of these other symptoms. Most all of them began immediately following my second surgery, although a few did develop and/or worsen in the months to follow. These I will call IC-related symptoms. I call them IC-related for two reasons. First, because I never had any of these symptoms prior to getting IC. And second, because these symptoms are commonly found in IC patients. They are much more common than you would think after reading all the IC literature, as most are rarely discussed. Many IC patients feel like they are "crazy" and that they are the only ones who have these "other", "weird" symptoms. This is just not so. I know hundreds and hundreds of IC patients and these symptoms are common. Not only does it add to the confusion when searching for a diagnosis, but also these symptoms are not being addressed by much of the IC research. I want you to know that you are not crazy if you have any, or all, of the following symptoms. (Personally, I had all the following symptoms except incontinence, canker sores, endometriosis, TMJ, Chronic Fatigue Syndrome, and Lupus.)

**Bladder** - Pain in the bladder that intensifies as the bladder fills and sometimes lessens upon voiding (for some), bladder pain immediately following urination, mild to extreme urgency, mild to extreme frequency (up to 85 or 100 times a day in severe cases), inability to start the urine stream, burning pain, burning during urination, cramping with sharp or shooting pains, urethra pain, blood in urine, mucous in urine, dark and/or cloudy urine, small pieces of tissue with blood attached visible in urine, bubbles in the urine, strong odor to the urine, recurrent "standard" bladder infections or urinary tract infections (UTI's), incontinence, reduced bladder capacity

**Kidneys** - recurring kidney infections, kidney inflammation and flank pain, burning pain and soreness in the kidneys, recurring kidney stones

**Teeth** - infections of the teeth and gums, mouth sores, canker sores, (a common site is the corners of the mouth), TMJ and/or jaw pain, sore tongue, burning tongue

**Allergies** - food and environmental allergies, sensitivity to medications (synthetic and natural), extreme chemical sensitivities

**Digestive problems** - acid stomach, (sometimes stomach ulcers or acid reflux), diarrhea and/or constipation, or one or the other, pain during bowel movements (Irritable Bowel Syndrome)

Nausea (increased when urine is held too long)

Pain, redness, swelling, itching, and severe irritation of the tissues covering the vaginal or vulva area (Vulvodynia)

Recurrent vaginal yeast infections and/or thrush (Candida)

Muscular and skeletal system problems - pain in all muscles and joints (Fibromyalgia)

Earaches, sore throats, sinus infections or sinus problems, lung congestion

Low-grade fevers every day

Low blood pressure (though some have high blood pressure)

Swollen glands all over the body (especially top of legs in groin area, throughout the neck and chest, and under arms)

Inflamed spleen and liver

Pain at the base of the neck

Itching with no rash present

Very accentuated PMS symptoms...extreme bloating, extremely painful cramps, heavy bleeding (blood clots), and irregular cycle. (All IC symptoms increase around menstrual cycle)

Migraines and/or severe headaches

Hypothyroidism (though some have hyperthyroidism)

Dry skin, dry hair, dry mouth, dry eyes (Sjogren's Syndrome)
Nerve pain down back of legs and/or arms
Bloating in pelvic area (e.g., looking like you're three months pregnant) and/or edema (swelling all over the body)
Inability to lie on left side (or right side) hip and leg
Night sweats and/or lack of perspiration
Unable to have anything touching pelvic area (clothes) due to pain
Sensitivity to bright light (painful to eyes)
Cold hands and feet (nose and ears) (Raynaud's Phenomenon)
Inability to tolerate extreme temperature changes
"Catching everything that's going around" (lowered immune system)
Lower back pain (can shoot up into the kidneys and/or down into the thighs)

**Associated Illnesses** (Many IC patients are also diagnosed with the following, the first four being extremely common.)
Fibromyalgia
Irritable Bowel Syndrome
Vulvodynia
Systemic candida infection
Sjogren's Syndrome
Raynauds Phenomenon
Migraines
Anemia
Mitral Valve Prolapse (MVP)
Endometriosis/cysts/fibroids
Chronic Fatigue (and Immune Deficiency) Syndrome
Systemic Lupus Erythematosus

Now obviously not every IC patient has every single one of these symptoms. (Though I definitely know some who come close. And I know I certainly did.) Also, I am not saying that if you have IC that you will necessarily develop every one of these symptoms and/or associated illnesses. But maybe you have some of the above symptoms and have never associated them with your IC. Or maybe you have associated them with your IC, but your doctor doesn't recognize the connection. And therefore maybe you are treating them all like they are separate diseases. Possibly you have the symptoms of some of the associated illnesses, but never went to get formally diagnosed. I know a lot of IC patients who have symptoms of Fibromyalgia or Vulvodynia, for example, but have not been formally diagnosed for various reasons. Whatever the case may be, if you have IC, especially a moderate to severe case, you most likely recognize that it is affecting the rest of your body as well. IC is not just a bladder disease. In my opinion, it can and will (if not treated) affect the entire body. I have experienced this myself and see it in other IC patients all the time.

# Chapter 6

———◆———

# Available Treatments

"Of the action of drugs we know little; yet we put them into
bodies about which we know less, to cure disease of which we
know nothing at all."
- Sir William Osler, MD

Here are the treatment options currently being offered by the medical
community for Interstitial Cystitis.

Bladder Distention:  The bladder is stretched to capacity by filling it
with water under general anesthesia. Many doctors claim that this
alleviates symptoms in some IC patients...to the point where they
actually refer to it as a "treatment". Personally, I don't know very many
IC patients who feel this way. It seems that the worse your bladder is
at the time of distention, the more likely it is that this procedure will
cause pain afterward and the less likely you will see much in the way
of "therapeutic" results. Many IC patients write to me asking if it's
normal to still be in a lot of pain a week or two after their
cystoscopy/distention. The answer, of course, is yes. It is definitely not
unusual. Actually, I have trouble understanding how stretching the
bladder to capacity in order to accentuate the cracking, bleeding,
and/or ulcers can be considered a therapy. To me this would be akin
to stretching the inside of the stomach to capacity in order to view
stomach ulcers or having a big cut on your arm and pulling the skin
apart as far as it will go so that you can see it better. I can't imagine
someone considering this humane, let alone therapeutic. I think the

41

only reason they have considered it "therapeutic" to stretch a bleeding bladder to capacity is that for the rare few who have mild IC, this stretching somehow temporarily deadens or destroys feelings in the nerves that signal pain. Otherwise, personally, I don't get it.

Oral Medications: Anti-inflammatory drugs, anti-spasmodics (e.g., Levsin or Levbid), antihistamines (e.g., Vistaril, Atarax) , muscle relaxants, bladder coating drugs (e.g., Elmiron) , tricyclic anti-depressants (e.g., Elavil, Doxepin) , pain medication (e.g., Demerol, Motrin, Ultram)

Bladder Instillations: Medications instilled directly into the bladder via catheter. (IC patients that I know who have tried bladder instillations of any kind recommend that you ask for a pediatric size catheter.) Various medications are held in the bladder for various amounts of time. I have found that the amount of time depends upon the particular medication being instilled, as well as on the doctor who is instilling it.

DMSO (Dimethyl Sulfoxide), which used to be used as an industrial solvent and as a horse liniment, is FDA approved for use as a treatment for IC. Some doctors say that DMSO helps to reduce inflammation and pain because it seeps into the bladder lining. And others say that it's purpose is to burn the bladder lining with the hope that it will rebuild itself, similar to a bladder wash. The garlic smell, which seeps out of your pores following treatments, is one of the more pleasant side effects. I know several IC patients who have had their vision permanently affected by DMSO. Many say that it caused weight gain that they could not get rid of. I also know that a rash or flu-like symptoms following treatments are also not uncommon. Many say that it made their bladder much worse and that they would never do it again. (See survey in the Appendix.) However, I also know some IC patients who had no adverse effects from DMSO. And there are a few that say it helped them go into remission briefly,  but that it most certainly did not cure them. I also know a few people who had their leg/thigh permanently burned by the DMSO after it leaked out during a treatment. What does this tell you about what the DMSO is doing in the bladder? There are some compassionate doctors who first use some numbing medication before instilling DMSO to reduce pain and discomfort. And if you're lucky, your doctor will also provide some type of pain medication before the procedure. One IC patient I spoke to said that her doctor gave her an injection of Demerol twenty minutes prior to the instillation.

Silver Nitrate and Clorpactin WCS-90 (Oxychlorosene Sodium) are both medications that are typically used while the patient is under anesthesia because the treatment is so painful. These "medications" are used as a bladder wash to strip or burn the bladder lining. This is done based on the premise that there is a defect in the bladder lining. The treatment is done with the hope that the bladder lining will rebuild itself, and therefore, no longer be "defective". (I can barely stomach the idea that this "treatment" is still in use today.)

Heparin works to coat the damaged cells in the bladder lining. "They" say it should be instilled on a regular basis over a year to 18 months. You don't feel the results of the treatments right away. It takes a long time for the heparin to build up and coat your bladder lining. I know IC patients who self-catheterize at home with heparin in combination with other treatments.

Cystistat (hyaluronic acid) is currently approved for use in Canada, but not yet approved by the FDA in the US at the time of this writing. Hyaluronic acid is a naturally occurring glycosaminoglycan which is found in all the connective tissues of the body. Cystistat is believed to coat the bladder lining and is similar in that respect to Elmiron and Heparin. To find out

43

about trying Cystistat, you can have your doctor call Bioniche at 1-800-567-2028.

There are other types of bladder instillations as well, such as Marcaine/Sodium Bicarb solution or various combinations called "cocktails", which sometimes include steroids.

Elmiron - An oral bladder coating drug. Still new to the market, this drug has had a lot of hype. I know a lot of IC patients who cannot tolerate Elmiron. I do know of some who feel it has helped at least some of their IC symptoms. So far, I am not aware of anyone who has had long-term success with this drug, but I don't think it's been out long enough to know yet. Elmiron is another drug that you have to take for a period of time (3-6 months) before knowing if it's helping you or not. If it does work for you, you need to take it the rest of your life or your symptoms return. Some side effects that I've heard from IC patients include, but I'm sure are not limited to, severe headaches, rashes, stomach/intestinal upset, and clumps of their hair falling out. I know some IC patients on Elmiron who reduced their dosage to reduce and/or eliminate the side effects. Some people I know experienced an increase in their symptoms when taking Elmiron. (So don't think you're the only person this has happened to if this was your experience.)

Bladder Holding Protocol - This is where the patient tries to control the frequency of voiding. Using a voiding diary/schedule and relaxation techniques, the IC patient tries to control their frequency. Though I have heard of IC patients who say that this has helped them with their frequency, I would still caution against this approach unless your bladder is well on it's way to being healed. And then, in my opinion, you probably won't need it. Otherwise, (I can't help it) I just see it as another form of torture that IC patients are asked to endure. Somehow it seems to imply that we can control our frequency by sheer will power.

Bladder Massage - Used to relax the bladder muscles.

TENS Unit for pain - (Transcutaneous Electrical Nerve Stimulation) A special device is used to send mild electrical pulses to the bladder and suprapubic area. TENS is used to help with pain and frequency. It is said to help increase blood flow to the bladder and possibly help strengthen the pelvic muscles. Some of my friends who use TENS for pain say they can only use it for a couple days at a time before it's effects wear off and then they have to take a break from it for it to work again.

The IC Diet - I do not replicate the IC diet here because I have found that except for the basics, we are all different in what foods we can tolerate. (You can get a copy of the IC diet from the ICA or your doctor.) Basically, it is important to avoid the obvious IC no-no's. No alcohol, nothing spicy, no caffeine, no chocolate, no carbonated beverages, no citrus, no MSG, no artificial sweeteners like nutrasweet, nothing acidic like tomatoes, vinegar, or lemon juice. One of my favorite IC buddies uses the rule "if it tastes good, spit it out" as her IC diet. There are several people that I know of who are writing IC cookbooks, and I imagine that at least one will be available by the time this book is finished. (Many IC patients who also have Vulvodynia are also trying the low oxalate diet with some success.)

Laser surgery - Sometimes used on bladder ulcers.

Bladder removal - Typical of IC, this is yet another controversial treatment option. Usually seen as a last resort (thank goodness!).

Antibiotic Therapy - Also very controversial, this type of treatment is hotly debated among IC patients on a continual basis. (more about this later....)


None of these seem to be an ideal choice. You will find criticisms and benefits of specific treatments, as well as comments from other IC patients, in the questionnaire results in the Appendix.

*Strength in tears...*

# The Pain of IC

The pain of IC is so hard to explain
To a world full of people who so often place blame
On the victims of this and other disease
Where understanding is lacking; there's no knowledge to please

IC is a disease that no one can see
They want to blame you; they want to blame me
It's all in your head - they tell you at first
They tell you you're crazy, till you think you might burst

It's hard to get past the anger you feel
After doctors have told you - it's nothing that's "real"
When they finally get around to looking inside
Our bladders are raw - they can no longer deny

They finally believe you and know you're in pain
But cures they can't offer; only treatments in vain
With no cause and no cure, IC is no fun
It's painful and lonely - not much can be done
Though they're searching for answers every day
It's not all we can do - to hope and to pray
We must do much more than that  - you see
If we're going to rid our bodies of painful IC


Written by: CATH767 - December 1995

# Chapter 7

———————◆———————

# Dealing with Doctors

"Doctors cut, burn, and torture the sick, and then demand of them an undeserved fee for such services."
- Heraclitus, Greek Physician, 500 BC

Not only was I not alone in how I got IC, I was also not alone in how I was treated by the doctors. Throughout my nightmare of trying to get diagnosed, I found the mistreatment at the hands of doctors to be phenomenally stressful, degrading, and physically painful. And, of course, I thought it was just me that this was happening to. Now I know better. Please try not to take it personally if you have been treated by unkind, insensitive, rude doctors. You would be astounded to know how many of us are out here. It is definitely not you. You are not a "bad" patient. You are not crazy. And you are not causing yourself to have IC. You are not causing or imagining your symptoms.

I started out as many of you probably did, as an uninformed, trusting consumer of medicine. And this was just my first mistake. I was always trying to act like a good patient and do what the doctor told me. It never occurred to me not to listen to everything my doctor suggested. I had always considered them the experts. It never occurred to me that I would have an illness that doctors didn't understand. It also never occurred to me that I would *ever* be treated as if I were crazy or imagining my symptoms either. It was frustrating, stressful, and quite frankly, scary, trying to prove to the doctors that something was physically wrong with me.

Being a female had its drawbacks when looking for medical help. I was automatically viewed a certain way because I was a woman. This doesn't just happen with IC patients. It happens to a lot of women with other health problems as well. It is well known that more women die of heart attacks today because they are doubted when they arrive at the emergency room. They are assumed to be having some kind of anxiety attack or that their problem is emotional rather than physical. As a thin, young female, instead of being seen as physically ill, I was viewed as anorexic. And when they discovered I was dehydrated, they assumed that I was denying myself food and drink rather than looking for a physical cause.

When it comes to IC, we have another issue to deal with as well. The percentage of urologists who are male is very high; up in the ninetieth percentile. And as one of the urologists I saw told me, "Prostates are where the money is.". So being that most IC patients are women looking for help in a male dominated field that has traditionally studied male urology versus female urology problems, we are automatically in a disadvantaged situation. I know some people may think this situation has improved, but as far as I know (and I talk to IC patients from across the country almost daily), it remains the same today as it was three years ago when I was trying to get diagnosed. Tragically, IC patients are still being mistreated and misdiagnosed every single day.

The pre-judgment that many urologists make when looking at women with "unexplained" bladder symptoms is that it must be an emotional problem. The older urologists were actually taught this in medical school! I know one older male urologist in my area who has mistreated so many IC patients (and continues to do so to this day) that when he volunteered to speak at a local IC support group meeting, everyone refused to come. (This just so happens to be the same doctor who told me that prostates are where the money is, the same doctor who misdiagnosed me three times, the same doctor who told me I had emotional problems causing my bladder symptoms, the same doctor who poked me in my swelling and told me that maybe I just gained some weight, the same doctor who squeezed my inflamed, infected kidneys to show me where my kidneys were located, the same doctor who did an in-office cystoscopy and wouldn't stop when his nurse told him I was turning white. Same guy.) He is so hated by IC patients all over the city that I'm surprised he doesn't just drop over from the hate vibes sent his way. Actually, I'm surprised there aren't urologists all over the country that don't just drop over from the hate vibes sent to them from IC patients. That's how bad the mistreatment remains.

Sadly, there are many doctors (and nurses in doctor's offices) who have said things to IC patients like "I don't know why you keep coming back here when there is nothing that anybody can do for you." Or they say "we can't just keep prescribing pain medication to you over and over again". I have heard this on several occasions. As I mentioned earlier, there are still some doctors today who will tell patients that IC does not really exist. That it is really an emotional illness of women. And there are others, who, though they do believe IC exists, don't realize how bad it can be. Nor do they recognize the fact that it affects the entire body. Some doctors will admit the logic of the association between IC and other illnesses, since they very often see IC patients who have fibromyalgia and IBS, etc.. But since the researchers have not nailed down the exact connection yet, they will continue to claim that there is not an "official" connection. So they don't really tell you, the patient, about them. You just go around thinking that you're the only one.

There are many doctors (if not most) that are very insensitive to the pain of IC. Unfortunately, it is very common to hear of urologists refusing to prescribe pain medication to IC patients. This is definitely considered common practice when you speak to IC patients across the country. Urologists, very often, seem to consider themselves NOT in the business of prescribing pain medication. (I have no idea how urologists can claim to "treat" IC and at the same time tell you that they don't treat the pain, since this is very often a prevailing symptom of the disease. And yet this happens all the time.) Many IC patients I know go to pain clinics or pain doctors to treat their IC pain. Others have compassionate internists who will write them prescriptions. There are some, however, who actually have a urologist who treats their bladder pain. Though it is rare, it is not completely unheard of. If you have a doctor who will not prescribe you anything for the pain, *find a new doctor*. I know how difficult it can be to ask for pain medication, but just because your doctor does not understand IC, does not mean you should have to suffer.

It was my IC friends who told me that I didn't have to suffer without pain medication just because my doctor was ignorant about IC. They convinced me to find a new doctor who would address the pain. One of my new IC friends had given me the phone number of Dr. Daniel Brookoff, an oncologist familiar with IC pain, from Memphis, TN. In a moment of painful desperation, I actually called and spoke with him. I want to express my sincere thanks to Dr. Brookoff who, not knowing me from Adam, returned my phone call and spoke to me for almost half an hour. Not only that, but he offered to talk to my doctor (if I could find one) about getting me something for the pain. I never had to take him up on his offer, but I appreciated it more than he could know.

As I mentioned earlier, the last urologist I saw told me that I had to have bladder instillations or else he would give me nothing for the pain. The fact that invasive treatments were not MY first choice of treatments, after reviewing all my options, did not make this urologist too happy. (Some doctors don't like it when their patients actually research their options and then make decisions about their health and their own bodies all by themselves.) This doctor was not willing to "treat" me unless I was willing to follow his treatment protocol for IC. This is certainly not unusual. However, I do not mean to say that all urologists use bladder instillations as their first line of treatment. Or that all urologists are this closed-minded when it comes to alternative treatments for IC. If you have an open-minded urologist who is willing to explore alternatives with you, consider yourself blessed and lucky.

If you go to a doctor and he even hints that this is all in your head, obviously you should get a new doctor. If you go to a doctor and he refs to what you have as a syndrome, personally, I would get a new doctor. If you go to a doctor that you don't feel comfortable with, that doesn't listen to you, that doesn't answer your questions, *definitely* get a new doctor. It's a good idea to ask how many other IC patients your doctor has and what type of success he has had in treating them. It's an even better idea to try and speak with some of his or her patients.

I think we tend to forget, as patients, that we are the consumer when we go to the doctor. Don't forget that the doctor is working for you. If you are not happy with the service you are getting, you are free to go to another doctor. Also, please remember that you do not have to listen to and obey everything your doctor tells you. This is so important where IC is concerned as the treatments often have side effects and risks, not to mention that they are sometimes painful. Better to get advice, weigh all your options and make your own informed decisions where IC treatments are concerned.

Keep in mind that some doctors who are treating IC patients and/or who are considered "IC experts" are getting paid research dollars. In one respect, this is a really good thing, because, of course, we want doctors out there doing research on IC. However, you might want to check to see what type of research your doctor is doing, if any. Does he get money to research a specific IC treatment? Is this the treatment approach he is planning to use with you? Is it because this is his area of research or because this is what is best for you? Is he willing to listen about other treatment approaches that you might feel are better in your particular situation? (These are just some things to consider. Just some things to think about.)

Remember that doctors are human. And just like in any profession, there are some good ones and some lousy ones. What always puts it in perspective for me is to remember some of the idiots that I went to school with and how some of them grew up to become doctors. (Nice of me...huh?) Remember that many people go into medicine with dollar signs in front of them, rather than the noble idea of trying to help others heal. And yet, still we put them in charge of our health and well-being. I think we sometimes forget that they are just "doing their job" and that they are not required to care about us. Also, please keep in mind that "they" call it a medical industry for a reason. It is, after all, a business. And the goal is not always so lofty as the care of patients. I know you won't be surprised when I tell you that it is very often related more to financial goals.

At the same time, realize that as IC patients, we are no picnic for the medical doctor either. They very often do not understand our pain, frustration, desperation or fear. Plus, and more importantly, they don't know what to do for us. Therefore, to them, I believe, we are very often considered a "pain in the neck".

At first, after getting diagnosed with IC, I was in a panic trying to find a urologist. After all, I *did* have a bladder disease. It seemed only logical that I go to a specialist. It sure seemed like the right thing to do. Actually, I thought I *needed* one. Even after all the horrendous experiences I had just had, I still thought I didn't have a choice but to find a doctor. Not only that, but I actually searched for an "IC expert", thinking this was the only way I was going to get better. At one point, I was even willing to fly across the country to see a urologist who was considered an "IC expert", though I never did. And I never found a urologist to treat my IC either. As it turns out, for me, this was probably the best thing that could have ever happened.

I understand that many who will read these words are very much into the medical "ideas" and treatments about IC. I know that most of the IC patients I speak with believe the doctors (and the medical community) when they are told that IC is incurable. They believe that their only options are those offered by the medical community (or their doctor) and that they must "learn to live" with their IC. Maybe you believe this too. Maybe you have been offered "self-help techniques" or told to keep a positive attitude and be "pro-active" as a patient. Maybe you have no idea what that really means. Maybe you think that's just another way of saying "learn to live with it". Maybe some of you are at the point right now where you believe that all there is left to do is to treat the pain. Maybe you have a morphine pump already, or a TENS, or maybe you're thinking about getting a nerve block. Maybe you are completely and totally depressed because you just can't imagine the rest of your life like this. Well, I am here to tell you that you don't have to live the rest of your life like this. You do not have to have IC forever. You don't have to just "learn to live with it". There ARE other things to try. There are...alternatives.

# Chapter 8

───────◆───────

# Why consider alternatives?

"Neither ought you to attempt to cure the body without the soul; for the reason why the cure of many diseases is unknown to the physicians....is because they are ignorant of the whole, which ought to be studied also, for the part can never be well unless the whole is well."
- Plato

First of all, I certainly don't want to discount the usefulness of doctors or the medical profession. Obviously, medical doctors are wonderful for surgeries and emergencies. I mean, if I were having a heart attack or needed my arm sewn back on after a car accident or something, I would definitely want a medical doctor and/or surgeon. No question about it. But medical doctors are not so great, and admittedly so, at treating chronic illness. There are many chronic illnesses that medical doctors do not understand or know how to treat. IC is only one of them. However, whether they have a clue about IC or not, I do believe it is a good idea to align yourself with at least one good doctor. One who believes in you, listens to you, and is willing to look at alternatives. And most importantly, one who will write you prescriptions when you need them. To be perfectly honest, this was my main reason for having one.

Now...why consider alternative treatments when it comes to IC? 1) Doctors, on the whole, have very little understanding of IC...and they tell you this. 2) They offer invasive, often painful, treatments or medications, none of which, and they tell you this too...work for everyone. (Typically, not even 50% of the people who try them get relief.) 3) The treatments and medications they do offer may possibly do more harm than good...and they very often don't tell you this. 4) The medical community has not yet identified (or agreed upon) a cause for IC and hence are "making it up as they go along", in terms of treatment, with IC patients as their guinea pigs. They call it a medical "practice" for a reason. They are definitely *practicing* on IC patients. Just as most doctors today consider urethral dilations to be barbaric, I believe that most of the IC treatments of today will someday be viewed the same way.

Modern medicine provides many quick fixes. They offer pills that often cover symptoms almost instantaneously. But curing or healing does not always take place. And then more medication is needed. Stronger medications, different medications, or just more medications. Eventually more problems will arise because the "cause" is not being addressed, the symptoms were just suppressed. I believe this is the case with IC. There is obviously more to IC than the medical community, at this point, recognizes or understands. It is my belief that they are very often hurting, rather than helping, the IC patient.

I do realize that there are some IC patients who truly like their doctors and trust them, which is wonderful. But there are also many of us who have had terrible experiences with doctors. Too many of us have been mistreated, physically hurt, insulted, and told stupid things by doctors. Me...well...I was grateful to have alternatives.

Typical of mainstream medicine, most IC treatments are geared toward covering symptoms. A variety of approaches are used with the hope that one of them might alleviate symptoms and that somehow, often mysteriously, the patient will go into remission. For example, bladder instillations are used to either 1) numb the nerves to the bladder to reduce or cover-up symptoms, 2) coat the bladder lining to reduce or cover-up symptoms, or 3) burn the bladder lining with the hope that it will rebuild itself "healthier". This is all based on the premise that the bladder is the problem. *Mainstream medicine's approach to IC has been to forget that the bladder is attached to the rest of the body.* Evidence of this lies in the treatments and in the fact that urologists are still the ones treating IC.

Just as I would recommend not to listen to everything your doctor tells you, based on the above, without thorough research on your part, I would also recommend the same if you are speaking to an herbologist, a naturopathic or holistic doctor, an acupuncturist, a psychic healer, or whoever. Get advice from your doctor or alternative healer, but know that you don't have to listen to everything they tell you. *Trust yourself instead.* Get advice and then do some research before making your decisions. Because they *are* your decisions. If you are going to take herbs, for example, check out information on the particular herb from many different sources. Do not just read one book, read three. Do not take just one person's word alone. Mine included. Make sure you listen to your gut feelings and to what feels right to you. This is very important. Talk to other IC patients (most importantly) and research, research, research before trying anything. Because with IC, there are no easy answers.

Personally, I did not have a lot of success with the first couple alternative treatments I tried. For example, the very first thing I tried after getting diagnosed was acupuncture. I had met a couple of IC patients on line who were using acupuncture with some success. I had also read that even mainstream medicine was recognizing that some IC patients were finding relief through acupuncture. This had me hopeful and I thought I would give it a shot. When I did, however, I had a lot of trouble staying on the table because of my frequency/urgency. It was $95 a treatment and of course was not covered by my insurance. It may have been worth the effort and money if I could have at least stayed on the table with the needles for more than 5 minutes at a time. Every time the doctor got all the needles in place, I would have to get up to go to the bathroom. So he would have to take them all out, I would get dressed, walk down the hall to the bathroom....and by the time I got back, undressed, and got back on the table.....I would have to go again. You know how it is. (Who's kidding who? You know I had to go before I even made it out of the bathroom.) I do remember that it helped some though. The little bit I was able to do. I think it would have helped more if I had gone later when my frequency was not as out of control. This was not as big a mistake as the next alternative thing I tried.

I went to an herbologist who insisted that it didn't matter what IC was. Every time I tried to tell her what it was, she cut me off and said it didn't matter. She said that she could test me for vitamins and herbs and that somehow my body would tell her what it needed. She used some form of applied kinesiology or muscle testing. She also told me that the bladder represented anger and that I must have been angry or "pissed off" at my dad for dying and that this was the reason I was sick. I totally disagreed with her of course. I may have been angry, but it certainly wasn't at my dad. I didn't argue with her though. Partly because I didn't really care much what she thought and partly because all I could think about was that I had to go to the bathroom. Actually, I remember that she noticed that I went to the bathroom a couple of times and then there was ten minutes or so where I hadn't gotten up to go. She told me she thought it was psychological about "why" I had to go. I also totally disagreed with that, of course. As you probably know, there are times with IC where your bladder spasms and "freezes up" and you just can't go because nothing will come out. (One of my IC friends calls this "pee freeze".) That was what was happening. So for those ten minutes, I was just trying to "hang in there" and get through this appointment. She just had no idea, of course, which is my main point here. She had absolutely no idea what IC was or what it was about. She may have known a lot about vitamins and herbs, but she knew nothing about IC. Yet here she was giving me advice about it anyway. Which is fine I suppose, as long as I didn't listen. It was my decision to listen to her. *I have since learned never to listen to someone tell me what to take who doesn't understand IC.* This includes doctors, healers, herbologists or whoever. But, that afternoon, I ended up getting a couple hundred dollars worth of vitamins and herbs. Whether

I agreed with the rest of what this woman said to me or not, I did not find it that difficult to believe that my body needed the extra nutrition.

The next day I did one of those stupid things that I'm hoping I can get you to avoid. I took a whole handful of these various herbs and vitamins in the dosage the lady had recommended. I had a huge, horrible, terribly scary reaction. It was like toxic overload or as if I had been poisoned. The bladder pain this caused was just insane and completely indescribable. And the rest of my body didn't react very well either. It took two to three days for it to get out of my system and for me to get back to my "normal" pain levels. My bladder was bleeding like crazy from this stupid "experiment". My stomach and intestines went nuts. Even if my body did need all this nutrition, my bladder definitely couldn't handle it at all. Neither could the rest of my body. This was a major lesson for me.

As IC patients, we are very vulnerable. Because we are so desperate to get well, we often fall prey to scams and can easily get manipulated into buying all kinds of "remedies" to make us well. *Believe me...everyone will be trying to sell you something.* Even well meaning people can easily hurt us. This is the tricky part. Even though they don't understand IC, they will most assuredly offer advice anyway. They may know a lot about their particular form of alternative therapy, but they still may not realize the extreme sensitivities of an IC patient. *You will have to decide when to listen.* There are tons of different "alternative" treatments out there. And though I believe that "alternative" treatments are the way to go with IC, you really have to be very careful and discerning. Just because something is "all natural" does not mean that it can't hurt you. And just because someone knows a lot about herbs and vitamins does not mean that they know how to "prescribe" them for an IC patient.

*A Healing Path...*

# Chapter 9

---◆---

# What exactly did I do?

*"Let every eye negotiate for itself, and trust no agent."*
*- Shakespeare*

Getting well, for me, has not been straightforward. It very often seemed to be "two steps forward, one step back". Keeping the faith during the small and large setbacks along the way certainly wasn't easy, but I found it almost essential to my healing that I continued to believe that I would get well. I want you to believe that you can get well too. I want you to believe it, because it's true. And because it's important in your healing. As awful as they were, my setbacks often led to more answers and greater understanding.

Most IC patients that I talk to ask me the same question. They all want to know *exactly* what I did to get better. I always wish that I could give a simple answer. But the answer, unfortunately, isn't so simple. It takes many different things to get rid of IC. Because IC is many things. And it also takes time. In sharing what treatments I've tried and what worked for me, please don't think that the same exact "prescription" will necessarily work for you. This is very important. We are all at a different place with our IC. What was appropriate for me at a given time, may not be something you would want to do in your given circumstances. Not to mention that I most certainly made some mistakes along the way. At the same time, I'm hoping that by briefly describing what happened to me and what I did, it may help you to better understand your IC and your treatment choices as well.

There were several reasons that I chose the antibiotic therapy as my first (and as it turned out...only) "medical" treatment. I believed from the start that my IC was directly related to my surgery and to my subsequent bladder/kidney infection. (How could I not? I woke up with symptoms that I didn't have before they put me under.) There was also the fact that they had found all kinds of bacteria in my urine following the surgery that was not there before the surgery. My other symptoms all seemed to point toward infection (e.g., the low grade fevers every day, swollen spleen, bleeding bladder, the swollen glands all over my body). And, I should also add, in order to be perfectly honest, that I was very much against trying any invasive treatments after what I had already been through. Since I believed I got IC from the surgery/catheter in the first place, and after my "catheter nightmare", I wanted nothing to do with another catheter if I could help it. For all of these reasons, antibiotics seemed like a good option for me at the time.

Through my IC friends on line, I discovered the work of Dr. Paul Fugazzotto. I spoke to several other IC patients who were undergoing his antibiotic treatment. I also spoke to IC patients who were on antibiotics with Dr. Durier and Dr. Dominique. Dr. John Warner, an infectious disease doctor at the University of Maryland and Dr. Stewart Weg from Philadelphia are also among those that argue that there is a bacterial connection with IC. I was aware of their work as well.

Even at this point in my discussions with other IC patients, I learned enough to know that the ones who were going through bladder instillations, on the whole, were not getting any better. The statistics you are given by your doctor simply do not reflect what you will find yourself when you speak to other IC patients. Even at this early stage, I recognized that the majority of IC treatments were directed only at the bladder. I knew there was more to it than that. I knew I wasn't the only one who had other symptoms throughout my body. And since my thinking at this point was that IC was an infection of some kind, I decided to call Dr. Fugazzotto and have him do a culture.

68

Dr. Paul Fugazzotto has been a pathogenic microbiologist for over sixty years. At the time that I went on antibiotics under his direction back in November 1995, he had well over 1500 IC patients across the US and in Canada. Dr. Fugazzotto argues that the culturing techniques used by most hospitals and doctors office labs are not sophisticated enough to detect the bacteria in IC patients. Instead of the typical plate culture that determines infection based on a colony count, Dr. Fugazzotto uses a broth culture technique to help him isolate bacteria in the urine samples of IC patients. Another difference is that most cultures are grown for 2-3 days, which is, according to Dr. Fugazzotto, not a long enough time for the particular bacteria that he finds in IC patients. Dr. Fugazzotto grows his cultures for 5-7 days. He believes that just because the bacteria doesn't grow in the typically allotted 2-3 day time period, doesn't mean the patient isn't sick. One of the times I spoke to him on the phone, he told me how the culturing method being used today has never been scientifically tested and was right out of Biology 101. It is highly outdated and he refers to it as a "Mickey Mouse" culture.

My culture showed enterococcus, which is one of the more common, but not the only, bacteria found in IC patients Dr. Fugazzatto tests. He recommended specific antibiotics after doing sensitivity tests against the bacteria. For me, he recommended Augmentin, which turned out to be too strong. It actually caused more pain and discomfort with too much antibiotic in my system, so he switched me to 250mg of Augmentin and 500mg of Amoxicillan a day. The combination worked better. I stayed on antibiotics for four months, during which time the bleeding from my bladder subsided tremendously. I went from large blood clots and bleeding between and during urination, down to a small amount of blood in the urine. For me, this was a big improvement. The pain, frequency and urgency were all reduced, and for the first time, I thought I was heading toward remission. However, I was still having several other symptoms and some were actually getting worse (e.g., the muscle/joint pain, the swollen glands). I still had a swollen belly and pain in my bladder at this point. My frequency and urgency were better than before, but still remained.

Back in 1995, there was a whole group of us on line who tried antibiotics under the direction of either Dr. Fugazzotto, Dr. Durier, or Dr. Dominique. As I recall, most of the people I knew did have improvements on the antibiotics. Though there were a couple who felt they made them worse. And many people who saw improvements in their symptoms had to eventually get off of the antibiotics because of the side effects they were experiencing. I'm not referring to the stomach upset typically associated with antibiotics, but rather a seriously lowered immune system or severe intestinal problems. Long-term antibiotic therapy is certainly not without risks. There can be serious repercussions.

Recognizing the dangers of long-term antibiotics and wanting to get off of them as soon as possible, I searched for an alternative. Antibiotics definitely take their toll on your immune system and they also prime the body for yeast overgrowth; killing not only the "bad" bacteria, but the "good" bacteria as well. Dr. Fugazzotto had found yeast in a couple of my samples and had recommended Diflucan as an anti-fungal medication. Each time, after taking Diflucan, I noticed I would feel somewhat better. It was at this point that I started reading and researching about systemic candida (systemic meaning all over the body and candida meaning yeast). I was beginning to realize that yeast was definitely part of the problem for me. I did not see it as "the" cause of my IC, just that it was present and was an issue to be dealt with. The more I learned about systemic candida, the more I realized the role it plays in IC. Though I am certainly not an expert on candida, I will briefly explain systemic candida hoping that you will read more about it elsewhere.

### What is Systemic Candida?
Yeast live in and on our bodies from the moment we are born into this world. It is normal to have yeast in the body. What is not normal is to have an overgrowth of yeast. Infection or any illness, physical or mental stress, lack of sleep, and/or poor nutrition all weaken the immune system and make us more

susceptible to yeast overgrowth. Medications such as steroids, antibiotics, and birth control pills can upset the body's balance, allowing yeast to thrive. Even the hormonal changes of pregnancy can throw the body enough out of balance that yeast can become a problem. Evidence of this is the fact that vaginal yeast infections are relatively common among pregnant women. There are many different things that can throw the body out of balance and provide a great environment for yeast to thrive.

When the yeast that normally live in the intestines and digestive system grow out of control, they begin to spread to other parts of the body. Once there is an overgrowth, the yeast changes form.  It changes into a fungal state where it produces over 75 known toxic substances and releases them into the body. These toxins enter the bloodstream and travel to various parts of the body. Therefore, yeast can cause a variety of health problems throughout the body. (You need not necessarily have a vaginal yeast infection to have systemic candida. Though getting vaginal yeast infections is very often a reflection that yeast is a problem systemically as well.)

I remember getting on line and talking to other IC patients about candida. I think they thought I was a little nuts at first (this was a few years ago). It took me a while to convince anyone to even read about it. As there were a number of us on antibiotics at the time, eventually others starting looking into it as well. Now, two years later, it appears that some type of anti-candida program is being recommended for those people trying antibiotics as a treatment for their IC. I am so happy to see this has become more accepted and somewhat standard practice. Because if you plan to take antibiotics (even short-term) you need to be careful of yeast overgrowth. This is true for "normal", "healthy" people, but especially if you have IC and are treating your IC with antibiotics. Not only that, but I have since found that whether you have mild, moderate or severe IC, candida most often still plays a role (whether you are currently taking antibiotics or not).

71

Diflucan is an oral medication that is intended for use as a one dose treatment for vaginal yeast infections. It was helping, but it wasn't enough. I was also concerned about taking it too often. I remember hearing something about liver damage associated with overuse. Realizing that traditional medicine rarely recognizes or treats systemic candida, I turned to alternative treatments.

It was at this point in my search that I came across an anti-candida program that I thought would be appropriate for me. It included several products, one of them being colloidal silver. This was the first I had heard of colloidal silver. Colloidal silver is considered to be both a natural antibiotic and an anti-fungal, so I thought it would work on both the "IC bacteria" and the candida. Before trying the colloidal silver, I did a lot of research. I was looking for medical evidence that colloidal silver was effective. It was very confusing because there were so many MLM (multi-level marketing) companies that were trying to sell the stuff. MLM's always make products look like a scam to me for some reason. There were so many brands out there and they all had a different amount of ppm's (or parts per million) of silver. It was difficult to decide whether or not to try this controversial product. Deciding whether or not to send a urine sample to Dr. Fugazzotto to see if he found bacteria was not as difficult a decision as deciding to try colloidal silver.

This was one of the many, many times that it felt like I was all on my own trying to figure out what to do, in terms of treating my IC. I later realized that I was basically always on my own in deciding what to do. No matter what, it was my body and I was the one who ultimately had to decide. However, the loneliness and scariness of being my own doctor is definitely something I became familiar with these past few years. It was a struggle sometimes to have faith in my own judgment and my own ability to research and make decisions that would affect my pain levels and my quality of life. These were not decisions to take lightly.

It was risky to try colloidal silver and though I experienced no negative side effects that I am aware of (and this is almost two years later), I am not necessarily recommending it. The reason being that I have since discovered other things that I would probably recommend more. If you decide that candida plays a role in your IC, there are many anti-candida products on the market to choose from. You really have to do your own research and feel comfortable with the products you choose.

It may sound silly, but when I read the booklet on the anti-candida program I eventually decided to use, I felt really good about it. I just "had a feeling" it was the right thing for me to do next. I called the director of the wellness center that used this program and spoke to him at great length about colloidal silver, as well as about candida and IC. I knew it was risky, but then, so was staying on the antibiotics. I ended up doing the anti-candida program for the next several months (3-4 months on the silver, 2-3 months or so on other anti-candida supplements, and actually continued on acidophilus for the next couple years).

I also called and spoke with Dr. Fugazzotto about colloidal silver before I got started. He agreed to test me after I took the colloidal silver to see if it was working. I was grateful for his open-mindedness and glad that he had at least heard of colloidal silver being used as an antibiotic. Dr. Fugazzotto did find anti-bacterial action in my sample, but not what he considered to be enough to kill the bacteria. Naturally, he recommended that I get back on the synthetic antibiotics. Not wanting to go back on the synthetic antibiotics because of what they were doing to my body, I increased the silver dosage instead.

Getting off the synthetic antibiotics was the big turning point for me switching over to all natural treatments. This was when I really became on my own. I was treating myself without the help of any doctor, without anyone telling me a specific dosage or length of treatment. And it seemed to be working. I was definitely getting better. The anti-candida program did reduce and/or eliminate many of my symptoms. My belly was flat again. My pain, frequency, and urgency were further reduced. And many of my "other" symptoms like swollen glands and muscle/joint pain had improved as well. For the second time, I thought I was heading toward remission.

During this time, I was continuing to treat my IC as if it were a systemic infection, without using synthetic antibiotics. Even though the exact bacteria had not been identified, I still saw a lot of evidence that made bacteria seem a logical choice as "the cause". At least for me, at this point, I felt it was the cause.

Shortly after getting diagnosed I remember hearing about a man who discovered that stomach ulcers were caused by bacteria. After decades of believing that stomach ulcers were caused by stress, this man proved that they were caused by a previously unidentified bacteria. He did this by giving himself the bacteria and causing himself to get an ulcer, and then curing himself of that ulcer. Many of us on line discussed the likelihood that IC would someday be discovered to be bacteria related. Bacteria causing ulcers in the stomach is not a far cry away from bacteria causing ulcers in the bladder. So if you're reading this book thinking that there is no way that IC is caused by bacteria because the doctors/researchers say so, you might want to consider that it wouldn't be the first time "they" were mistaken.

Antibiotics were helping a lot of people I knew at the time. They had helped me. There were, however, IC patients that were not being helped by antibiotics. Whether they couldn't tolerate the antibiotics or whether they were made worse by taking them, at the time I attributed to the candida factor. Especially for IC patients who had taken antibiotics repeatedly in the past and who probably already had systemic candida (in my opinion) prior to trying them again. It made sense to me that antibiotics would make them worse. But if IC *were* caused by bacteria, why had "they" not been able to identify it yet?

There could be a lot of reasons for that I suppose. Maybe IC is caused by a cell-wall deficient bacteria making it difficult to find. Maybe it is so microscopic that we just don't have the technology to see it yet. Though if this were the case, why would antibiotics not cure everyone? Was the candida getting in the way? Was it that the IC bacteria is so mutated and so antibiotic-resistant that it is just not so easy to kill? That is what many people who believe in the bacteria theory think. That IC is caused by a mutated, antibiotic resistant bacteria. And it very well may be. The jury is still out. But I can tell you one thing, it is definitely not difficult to find medical articles on nosocomial infections (infections acquired in the hospital) or the overuse of antibiotics and the increase of antibiotic-resistant bacteria. With so many people getting IC in the hospital and following repeated bladder infections, it doesn't seem so absurd to think that someday IC will be found to be bacteria related.

The bacteria theory is an incredibly controversial topic among IC patients. It has been hotly debated on line on several occasions. We all have our opinions and our experiences with antibiotics. Some would argue vehemently that if your IC was "cured" or helped by antibiotics, then you didn't have IC in the first place. That what you really had was a bladder infection. These are the people who agree with the current medical opinion of IC and believe that IC is not an infection. The reason that this is the "medical opinion" of IC is because it has yet to be proven that IC is caused by a specific bacteria. There are just as many IC patients who will argue (also vehemently) that IC is indeed an infection and that they were "cured" of their IC by taking antibiotics. I know IC patients who accidentally found that antibiotics helped their IC symptoms when they were taking them for something else. And I know others who tried antibiotics to treat their IC and experienced an increase in pain and symptoms. I know some IC patients who live on low dose antibiotics every day of their lives. It is the only thing that works for them. It is the only thing that holds their IC symptoms at bay. Interestingly, there are still others who believe the onset of their IC was due to antibiotics.

The research also reflects this controversy. For every research article that claims IC is not caused by bacteria, there is one that implies it might be. Statistics can be manipulated and results can be skewed. It is one reason that I chose not to quote research left and right in this book. It is for this reason also that I think you should read the research yourself and draw your own conclusions. Not to mention that the recent research of today, may not be so recent by the time you read this book. If there were the perfect IC study out there, that proved the cause or found the cure, I think we would all know about it by now. (And I'm quite sure I would be quoting it like crazy!)

# Chapter 10

———◆———

# How I see IC

Okay...so what is IC then? As I start to write this chapter I realize how difficult it is to write my opinions about IC. Everything about it is so controversial. Who am I to say what IC is? I'm obviously not a doctor or a research scientist. I am just an IC patient who got better. Maybe you will completely disagree with my opinions. That is okay. And if, in disagreeing, you understand your IC better, then this makes me happy. Looking at IC this way..."treating" it this way...is how I got well.

Obviously it is my belief that IC is not just a bladder disease. I don't think I know a single IC patient who got better by treating their bladder alone. I know many who have taken one medication or another and have gone into temporary remissions, but their IC always returns. A few have stopped their bladders from having any symptoms, but they are still not "healthy" in other ways. They still have "IC related" symptoms. Or they still have to avoid eating certain things or doing certain things. Or maybe they still have to take one medication or another every day for the rest of their lives (e.g., Elmiron, antibiotics). The additional symptoms that IC patients experience all point to the fact that IC does not affect the bladder alone. It is also interesting to note that many of the women who have had their bladders removed still have IC pain and "IC related" symptoms. I know a couple IC patients who have a neo-bladder (surgically made with part of their intestines) and the IC returned to their new bladder as well.

My experience with IC is that it is a systemic infection that throws the body off balance in many ways. Whatever is weak within the body will become weaker. IC attacks the bladder first and then goes on to effect whatever is weak within the individual. It will vary among IC patients, because we all have different physical weaknesses. Not only will it vary because of our different weaknesses, but also because we all develop different allergies. So what may be an allergen for one IC patient, may not be for another. Therefore, we do not react the exact same way to medications, food, or our environment. I believe this is a partial reason for our different symptoms and our different reactions to treatments as well.

Very often (but not always) IC is caused by an initial attack on the bladder, whether by bacteria (previous infection) or invasion by a catheter. It can also be a slower, more gradual attack on the bladder such as with candida toxins eventually compromising the bladder enough to be susceptible to IC. Or it may also be that an allergic reaction to the catheter compromised the bladder, making it the perfect environment for the "IC bacteria" to take hold. I would think that the bladder or nerves to the bladder can even be compromised or weakened by a previous back injury. Very often the bladder is compromised in some way prior to the onset of IC.

I believe that IC patients have a toxic body. Actually, to me, we are the *epitome* of the toxic body. The more severe the IC, the more toxic the body. You may feel as if you are on chemical overload, that you have too much acid in your system. In your stomach, intestines, in your kidneys and bladder, acid is burning in your system. That is what IC feels like to me. I believe we are constantly processing tons of toxins/poison. Everybody, of course, to a different degree. But this is why we have inflamed spleens and swollen glands. This is why all of our eliminative organs are, or can be, affected. From our skin to our livers, not to mention our kidneys and urinary tract. Every organ that processes waste in our bodies is affected. I believe this is also why most of us become chemically sensitive and/or develop allergies. It is fairly well known that IC patients develop allergies. (Well…as much as anything about IC can be well known.) It is my opinion that our bodies

78

simply cannot take any more additional chemicals/poisons/toxins. Whether they come from food, the environment, or medications, it doesn't matter. We are very SENSITIVE. Does this sound familiar? Sensitive to medications, sensitive to light, sensitive to smells, sensitive to everything. All of the mucous membranes in the body are (or can be) affected. They are inflamed and irritated (e.g., the intestines, the mouth, the sinuses, the bladder). *The toxic body of an IC patient provides the perfect environment for bacteria and fungus to thrive.*


## IC and Bacteria

Bacteria may not be THE cause of IC, but it most certainly is a factor for many people. Whether or not a specific IC bacteria has been identified or not, it has been shown that IC patients typically have bacteria in their urine more often than healthy controls. In other words, IC patients seem to get more "typical" bladder infections than people without IC. Whether this is because our bladder linings are not "healthy" enough to flush off the bacteria (e.g., the leaky gut theory) or because bacteria is involved in the cause of IC has not been determined. I know that I never had a bladder infection in my life until I got IC. I know many people, myself included of course, who experienced an improvement in their IC symptoms with the use of antibiotics. But whether that was because it was suppressing or killing *THE* IC bacteria or whether it was killing "other" bacteria, we can't be sure. The antibiotics could also be acting as an anti-inflammatory (as some antibiotics do), so we can't be sure of this either. Also, certain antibiotics have a stimulatory or inhibitory effect on the immune system, which could also be a factor. I also know many IC patients who cannot tolerate antibiotics at all because of allergic reactions or because it wreaks havoc with their immune system. There is also the issue of candida as a reason why some people can't tolerate the antibiotics. So of course, this all makes it very confusing.

Yes I took antibiotics for my IC. And yes...I did, and still do, believe that a combination of bacteria and fungus (yeast) infections played a major role in my IC. However, my understanding of IC has changed and broadened over the time I was working to heal myself. As my symptoms changed and my experiences grew, my opinions about IC changed as well.

At first I believed that IC was a systemic infection, plain and simple. My belief was based in part on the basic assumption that bacteria cause disease. I later learned that the presence of bacteria does not necessarily determine disease. In other words, just because specific bacteria are present, does not necessarily mean a certain, specific disease will manifest.

Back in the late 1800's, Louis Pasteur came out with his controversial research on the germ theory of disease. He proposed, at that time, that diseases were due to an invasion from an outside germ organism. He described how each type of bacteria was responsible for creating its own specific type of disease or illness. With more research, however, Pasteur later abandoned this "germ theory of disease" and declared that bacteria are *not* the exact and primary cause of disease. He became convinced that the bacteria were secondary and that the disease came first. However, his earlier germ theory was unfortunately considered a great scientific advancement at the time, so his later research and future discovery was suppressed. Even though Pasteur himself proved the fallacy of his own germ theory of disease, the propaganda was already out there and accepted. This error has been perpetuated to this day.

Pasteur himself said, "The presence in the body of a pathogenic agent is not necessarily synonymous with infectious disease." [1] The example is often used about a stagnant pond. The mosquitoes and gnats that are typically found around a stagnant pond did not *cause* the pond to become stagnant. A stagnant pond just happens to be the perfect environment for the mosquitoes and other bugs to flourish. There is no question that certain bacteria are associated with specific diseases, but the big question is: are these bacteria the accompaniment of the disease or are they the cause? I believe this question lies at the heart of the IC bacteria debate.

The fact is that bacteria live in and on our bodies all the time. We breathe in all kinds of bacteria every time we take a breath. Basically, we are exposed to bacteria all the time. So why are we not sick all the time? It has long been thought that females get bladder infections more often then men on the simple basis of anatomy. Because our orifices are very close together, infections were often blamed on lack of hygiene. If it were as simple as "bacteria cause infection", every baby that ever sat in a dirty diaper would have gotten a bladder infection. Obviously other factors attribute to whether or not infection or disease will develop. The mere presence of bacteria does not necessarily determine the presence of disease. It is the case, rather, that many variables come into play to create infection or disease. This, I believe, is the case with IC.

For example, I know a lot of IC patients who, believing that IC was an infection, decided to have their spouses tested by Dr. Fugazzotto. They wanted to make sure they were not passing it back and forth to each other. I know several people whose spouses were found to have enterococcus, yet their spouse did not have any IC symptoms. Why is that? And why is it that when Dr. Susan Keay examined IC patients against healthy controls, she found bacteria present, not only in IC patients, but also in the healthy controls? Why is it that the same bacteria affect some people and not others? *A toxic body can change the form and function of bacteria.*

Pasteur also recognized that bacteria and fungus change their forms according to their environment. Not only does their form change, but their physiological function changes as well. So that possibly, a bacteria could live in the body and cause no harm, but with a change in the environment within the body, the bacteria could change its form and function and thus cause harm. Could it be that IC is caused by a bacteria that normally lives in the body and does no harm, but when the environment of the body changes, it causes a change in the bacteria, thus causing harm?

If it were true that bacteria cause disease then everyone would most certainly be sick all the time. But if our immune systems were strong enough to protect our bodies from "invasion" by these bacteria, then we would not get sick. Or we could say, as is the case with auto-immune disease, if our immune systems were reacting "normally", then we would not experience sickness. If our bodies (or immune systems) did not "view" the bacteria as "foreign" or an "enemy" then the body would not react as if it were infected. The strength of our immune system, obviously, has an impact on whether or not infection takes hold. And part of this strength is our body's ability to flush out the wastes and toxins so that they don't take up permanent residence. Part of the strength of our immune system lies in the health of our colon.

## IC and Candida

In order to properly eliminate the toxins and waste from our bodies, it is important to have healthy intestines and regular bowel movements. The health of our intestines is dependent in part upon the natural balance between the microorganisms that normally reside there. When the balance is upset and candida takes over, many different health problems can arise. When the intestines are not healthy and the body is not absorbing nutrition properly or eliminating waste properly, the immune system can easily become compromised. This is the case with candida. Not only is the body not absorbing necessary nutrients or eliminating toxins/wastes efficiently, but also candida, in its fungal state, is releasing toxins and poisons into the body. All of this makes for quite a toxic environment.

I think that the issue of candida has been overlooked by mainstream medicine in general, let alone regarding IC. Medical doctors typically see candida infections as something that only AIDS or other severely immuno-suppressed patients get. (Not to mention, most doctors don't even consider IC patients as having a suppressed immune system.) It is extremely rare to find an internist or a urologist who will even consider candida as part of the problem (let alone the whole problem), though it is known that candida infections can mimic IC bladder symptoms. They can cause frequency, urgency, and irritation to the inside of the bladder and outside tissues of the vagina. There is such a thing as "yeast cystitis". If you have a mild case of IC, I would recommend researching candida as a possible cause. There are some excellent books out there on candida, including *The Yeast Connection and The Woman* by William Crook, which even has a chapter on IC.

In ignoring candida as a possible cause or contributing factor to IC symptoms, I believe mainstream medicine is missing part of the problem. *Systemic candida can mimic IC because both release toxins and poisons into the body. Herein lies the similarity and the confusion.*

It is interesting to note that some IC patients attribute the onset of their IC symptoms with taking repeated antibiotics. I know Vulvodynia patients, IBS patients, and Fibromyalgia patients, who are not necessarily diagnosed with IC, who also attribute the onset of their illness to repeated antibiotics as well.

In the next couple years I was to learn that there are other factors that play a role in IC. It wasn't necessarily enough to take antibiotics or do an anti-candida program with the antibiotics. Though I do know some people who claim to have been cured of IC this way, oftentimes more is needed, because oftentimes more is involved.

# Chapter 11

◆

# An Uncharted Path

After finishing the anti-candida program and thinking again, for the second time, that I was heading toward remission, Charlie and I decided to get married. We had wanted to wait until I was feeling better so that we could enjoy it more (as you might imagine), but financially it just wasn't smart to wait. At this point I had already withdrawn my 401k and my cobra health benefits were running out. Being married meant that I could be on Charlie's insurance. Plus, at the rate I was going with the anti-candida program, we thought I would be well enough by the time the wedding came around. We flew to Arizona, where some of Charlie's family lives, to have the ceremony. We had a small "alternative" style wedding (I know you're surprised) with a short ceremony (another shocker). With the stress of traveling with IC and from the actual physical "work" of traveling, by the time we got home I had another setback.

This was when my kidneys got much worse. My kidneys had been affected from the beginning, with an infection immediately following the surgery. I had also passed kidney stones between the time I got IC and the time I was finally diagnosed. My kidneys had been infected and inflamed before with the IC, but this was somehow different. Now my kidneys were the prevailing painful symptom. There were several times that IC related symptoms caused more pain and more problems for me than the bladder symptoms.

For the next two years, there were several overlaps with so many of my symptoms that it gets very confusing to explain. (A mélange of symptoms that only an IC patient can understand.) I had several bouts with my kidneys, severe fibromyalgia, major problems with my teeth and gums, and often had severe flu and sinus/chest congestion. My spleen was inflamed and painful, my stomach was acid, and my IBS symptoms remained severe. My immune system was so suppressed and/or overworked, that it took literally 16 months for my stitches to heal and fall out from the last surgery I had. Throughout the past few years with my IC, with maybe the exception of a short break or two when I thought I was heading toward remission, I had huge swollen glands all over my body, joint and muscle pain all over my body, IBS symptoms, Vulvodynia symptoms, swelling in the abdomen (which then spread to the rest of my body), pain at the base of my neck, earaches, jaw pain, and sore throats, low grade fevers the first couple years changing to lower than normal body temperatures this past year. This, of course, was all on top of my bladder symptoms.

It was during this time when my kidneys became infected and inflamed that I really started learning about and experimenting with alternative treatments even more on my own. Initially I went to my internist. And, typical of IC, sometimes infection would show up and other times it wouldn't, even though my symptoms remained essentially the same. After all the work I had done with the candida cleanse, I didn't want the yeast to come right back. However, I also knew that a kidney infection can be serious, so I was also afraid *not* to take the antibiotics. It was a big dilemma trying to decide whether to take antibiotics again. In the end, my internist prescribed them, but I didn't take them. Instead I got some books on herbs and acupressure. I started reading more about alternative ways to treat infection.

I decided that I would do things to boost my immune system so that my body could fight the infection on its own. Knowing that acupuncture was difficult, I got a book and taught myself acupressure that I could do at home. I used pressure points for all kinds of things. For example, there are pressure points to help flush the lymph system, to release water retention, to reduce pain in muscles and joints, and to release chest congestion. These are just some of the ones I used fairly often. I like acupressure for several reasons. For one thing, you can do it yourself. It's not hard to do. And most importantly you can control the intensity. If you are doing a flush, for example, and you start to feel completely awful, you just let go of the pressure point. It's that simple. You can go at your own pace, which is a major plus for IC patients.

I also used reflexology (foot and hand massages) throughout the entire time I was sick. I say I "used" it even though Charlie did all the work. Even before we knew what we were doing (reflexology-wise) Charlie was giving me foot massages all the time to try to make me feel better. I learned to meditate and started reading about the mind/body/spirit connection. I took herbal baths to pull toxins out of my body. I learned about herbs to fight infection, herbs to soothe my insides, and herbs to boost my immune system. I drank herbal teas and took herbal tinctures. For months I drank an herbal nutrition drink that looked liked weeds floating in a glass of kool-aid. Actually, that's pretty much what it was. We called it "the weeds". (Creative aren't we?) And Charlie invented a homemade nutrition drink that I could drink twice a day. (If you have moderate to severe IC I'm sure you know what I mean when I tell you that putting any significant amount of food in the stomach adds to the pressure and pain in the entire abdominal/pelvic area. So twice a day I would drink my nutrition instead and it would put less pressure on everything.) I went all out and even learned how to use crystals and color for healing. I will tell you more about all of this in the chapter about alternative treatments you can try at home.

The severe kidney problems went on for about a year. During that time, among other things, I drank a lot of marshmallow root (and sometimes comfrey leaf) tea to soothe my kidneys and bladder. When my kidneys hurt a lot I would put a few drops of non-alcohol marshmallow root tincture under my tongue and Charlie would put a cool (not cold) washcloth right over my kidneys. Sometimes he would just blow cool air on them and that would help. For infection, I also took

Echinacea/Goldenseal in liquid form. I drank a lot of water to flush my system every day. I also took Cat's Claw (sometimes called Una de Gato) to boost my immune system. When I absolutely had to, I took Pyridium and/or Demerol for pain. And I constantly prayed to God that I was doing the right thing.

Just as my kidneys were getting a little better, my tailbone went out and my fibromyalgia nightmare began. (I had painful muscles and joints almost from the beginning with my IC, but this was much different.) The first time my tailbone went out it was from something as simple as stepping up onto a curb. Soon after, my hips on both sides, my shoulders, my neck, and my tailbone were all "going out" whenever I did anything even remotely strenuous.

With swelling, which quickly spread to the rest of my body, I was living on ice packs 24 hours a day for several weeks. This progressed quickly to the point where I could no longer open the front door. I could no longer walk down the stairs without holding on to Charlie's arm and the railing. Everything became a slow and painful process. I couldn't put on my own shoes and socks. I couldn't cross my ankles or legs and I couldn't sit cross-legged anymore. Lifting up a book became nearly impossible. I lost my mobility, strength, and flexibility. My shoulders would pop out of their socket or my hips would go out if I so much as picked up a coffee mug. Sometimes while I was sleeping, I would wake up from muscle spasms that were so bad that they would push my bones right out of their sockets. I had to do all kinds of stretching and self-adjustments to get the bones to go back in. For some of the adjustments I needed Charlie's help. Sometimes I would have to wake him up at 3:00 in the morning so that I could lie at the end of the bed on my stomach and he could lift up one of my legs at a time and cross it over my body to put my tailbone back in. Or I would hang my head over the edge of the bed and take deep breathes while Charlie put pressure on my shoulders to pop them back into the sockets. Then I would immediately ice and well…basically…try to stop crying. Often I knew the bones were back in place when I got the chills and a big poison rush immediately following an adjustment. Most of the time I wasn't sure if they were back in or not. The pain made it very confusing. Later I learned that if I picked up something like a cup or small paperback book, I could tell if my bones were back in place. If they weren't, the pain would be excruciating. If they were, the pain level stayed relatively the same. (Good trick…huh?)

Anyway, I felt I couldn't go to a doctor to help with these constant adjustments for several reasons. First, because they were constant and at all hours of the day and night. Secondly, it was a nightmare to ride in the car. Bladder pain and urgency aside, Charlie would turn the corner (like a normal person, not like a maniac race car driver or anything) and my hip would go out. Bumps along the road had me screaming out in pain. It was just nuts to go in the car. Secondly, I couldn't let anyone touch me. Everything hurt. My whole body was so swollen and fragile. The only person I would let near me was Charlie. He understood the pain I was in and was really gentle and careful. Even Charlie hurt me by accident sometimes. It wasn't his fault of course. Often it was the middle of the night and he would be half asleep, I would wake him up crying hysterically from the pain. These were insane times, as you might imagine. Other times he would rush home from work to help me. If my hip or tailbone went out in the afternoon, I would have to wait until Charlie got home from work to help me get it back in.

I had to do something. So at this point, Charlie and I became instant physical therapists and I started swimming for physical therapy. I was trying to strengthen my muscles and trying to get the toxins out of them through exercise. We also thought this would help with the swelling. Going to the pool was a whole production. Charlie would have to help me get dressed. I couldn't put on my shirt without his help or my shoulder would go out. He put on my shoes and socks for me because I couldn't bend over or pull my legs up high enough to reach. The first few times I went swimming all I could do was get into the pool, stand there and cry, and then get out. The water pressure of the pool was so painful. If there was anyone else in the pool, it was torture from the waves. This had Charlie, a normally sweet and gentle man, wanting to murder small children as he watched them splash around and cause me more agony. Charlie bought me a kick board and little by little I started to do laps. I had to start in the shallow end of the pool because I wasn't strong enough to tread water and my laps were only the width of the pool. Some people would see us and think that Charlie was teaching me how to swim because he would walk back and forth along the side of the pool cheering me on.

By the time we got back home I would be exhausted. I would have take a shower right away to get the chlorine (and whatever germs might have been in the pool) off of me. Charlie would have to help me undress, help me into the shower and help me back out. He had to do everything. I couldn't even get my towel off the towel rack or dry myself off. I would swell up even more right after swimming. But each time I would feel better once I got back on the ice packs in the bed. Besides helping to move toxins out of my muscles and body, it was often swimming that would help put my tailbone or hip back in. It was most tragic when my tailbone or hip would go back in during swimming, only to go out again on the car ride home.

But, little by little I grew stronger and eventually, after literally months of hard work, I was able to swim about 25 lengths in the pool. Most of these were with the kick board though, because with the huge swollen glands under my arms and the swelling in my upper body, I still couldn't use my arms much. I was still swollen all over, but I was getting stronger and a little more flexible. I also started walking for exercise. We lived across the street from a brand new shopping mall. During the winter it was the perfect place to go and walk. So on the days we didn't go to the pool, Charlie took me to the mall and he would walk with me.

I remember looking at a picture of the lymphatic system, which I'm sure I hadn't seen since college biology. I remember realizing that my swelling was worse where there were the most glands. I hadn't realized that we have glands throughout the chest and all over the pelvic area. I remember wondering why no one ever talks about this in regard to the swollen pelvic area so typical of IC.

Anyway, during this time, my teeth and gums problems got even worse. My gums were inflamed and my teeth were fragile, loose, and painful. My teeth were constantly "shifting" in my mouth as the swelling in my gums went up and down. It was difficult to chew anything even remotely hard. My gums were receding and bleeding and a blister mysteriously formed on the back of my throat. Several years before I got IC, I had accidentally been hit in the face with a baseball bat playing softball. The bat broke in half while someone was batting and it hit my face and broke my nose, many bones in my face, and several teeth. At this point I believed that the IC was affecting my mouth, because for me, this was a physical weakness from getting hit in the face years before. I knew that other IC patients had problems with their teeth and gums, so this was certainly not unheard of in the world of IC. I didn't really know what to do about it. It wasn't like my dentist had any idea why this was happening. Urologists don't understand IC, I certainly couldn't expect my dentist to. I found some alternative treatments to try on my teeth and gums. I used tea tree oil for infection and black walnut oil to nourish and strengthen my gums. I rinsed with baking soda and water constantly to neutralize the acid. This went on for months.

So at this point, I had pain in my kidneys and bladder, the IBS, the swelling and the muscle/joint pain and now some pretty severe problems with my teeth and gums. Still I was swimming, taking herbal baths, lying on ice packs and rinsing my mouth constantly. Then from seemingly out of nowhere I got the flu with severe chest congestion. I could barely breathe and it was really scary. This is finally what prompted me to quit smoking the rest of the way. I had already cut way down and now I finally decided to totally quit. So there I was lying on ice packs 24 hours a day, with the flu, swimming (with the flu), taking herbal baths and drinking herbal tea, rinsing my mouth about a billion times a day and quitting smoking all at the same time. Needless to say, I was not happy. Aside from when my bladder was bleeding huge blood clots and everyone thought I was some kind of emotional nut-case, I think this may have been my most tragic.

I tell you all this not to complain, but to show you that it has taken a lot of work for me to get better. It was not an easy path, the one I chose. I am quite sure that many people thought me stupid for not having a urologist to treat my IC. If not stupid, they certainly wondered how I was managing. I also know there are people out there that are in an even worse situation with their IC, but I wanted you to see that you can go from severe IC, severe Fibromyalgia, severe IBS, and all these other IC related symptoms and *still* you can get better. Not only that, but I know there are many people in areas where they cannot find a doctor knowledgeable about IC or they can't afford to or are not well enough to travel to see one and they are left feeling like there is nothing they can do. Even without a urologist, rheumatologist, gastroenterologist, gynecologist, etc....even without an "IC expert"...you can still get better. I am not saying don't get help or advice from these people; I am just saying that you can get better without them if you have to (or in spite of them, depending on your perspective). You do not have to give up or think that things will stay this way forever. If you take a look at your individual situation, there will be a lot of things that you can figure out, a lot that you can do to help yourself get well. I'm hoping this book will help you do that.

Throughout the past few years, I had to learn to listen to my body and pay attention to all kinds of things in order to figure out what to do. For example, while I was swollen and on ice packs I mysteriously got this huge rash on the back of my thighs. It looked like giant mosquito bites all over with swelling around them. It took us a couple weeks to figure out that it was the new bathroom cleaner that Charlie had used to clean the bathroom, including the toilet seat (where as you know I spent most of my time). I was having an allergic reaction to the chemical cleaner. Once we figured it out, the rash went away and we learned to clean with non-toxic, environmentally safe cleaners instead.

This got me started thinking about what had changed when the systemic swelling got so out of hand. We realized the only change was a new mattress. Ironically, we had bought a new mattress at the same time this had all started thinking this would make me more comfortable.

After realizing that was the only thing that had changed, I did a little research and learned that there are all kinds of chemicals in the mattress material and formaldehyde was one of them. (Formaldehyde is also in cigarettes.) So I started to read all about formaldehyde allergies and learned that, among other things, edema/swelling can be one of the symptoms. I also learned that it is not that uncommon for people to have an allergic reaction to a new mattress. I was pretty surprised because I had never even heard of that before. So we did all we could to cover up the mattress and even got a hypoallergenic mattress cover. It helped, but I was still having other chemical sensitivities and the swelling, for the most part, was still there. Though once we figured out the mattress connection, I no longer had to live on ice all the time.

I also noticed that it was when I quit smoking that even more hell broke loose. I had been a smoker for about ten or eleven years. I knew it was bad for me. Every smoker knows that. Somewhere inside me, I had always known that I wouldn't smoke forever. And I was always so healthy, that I wasn't really concerned about it. At least not concerned enough to warrant quitting. But once I got IC, I found myself thinking a lot more about how dumb it was to smoke. At the same time, I found some type of comfort in smoking and knew it would be difficult to quit. I continued to smoke the first couple years I had IC. I was home alone most of the time, on a bed or in the bathroom, unable to do much of anything, often in pain and very uncomfortable. Cigarettes were like a companion or a friend because they made me feel better. But after doing all these alternative things and working so hard to clear my body of toxins and poisons, I started realizing that smoking was putting toxins and poisons right back into my body. I finally had to face that I needed to quit and I started cutting down. When I finally did quit, everybody would ask me, "Oh don't you feel better now that you quit smoking?" And I would say "uh...no...not really". Actually, it made me much worse. Then I learned why. I never knew it was common to get really sick after you quit smoking.

When you quit smoking your immune system kicks in and starts trying to clean out your body. Cutting way down to get ready to quit is what brought about the huge bout with the flu when I could barely breathe. And then quitting completely threw my body even more off balance. With all the toxins and chemicals from the cigarettes trying to leave my body, I became even more chemically sensitive and developed even more allergies. I could no longer tolerate being around perfume, exhaust fumes, gasoline fumes, cigarette smoke, or anything like that. My throat would close up and I wouldn't be able to swallow or breathe. It was totally scary. These symptoms became pretty severe and I could no longer be around people or go out in public at all. I couldn't even stand to be in the apartment when the dishwasher was running because of the smell of the soap coming from the steam that seeped out of the dishwasher. I could no longer burn scented candles or handle the smell of body lotion. I could no longer walk at the mall because of the perfume smells. I couldn't believe how sensitive I had become. I began to realize that I had to do something about these allergies if I was to ever have any life at all.

I was lucky. Not only did coincidences lead me to an alternative doctor who practices NAET, but also her office was located right around the corner from our apartment. NAET is a technique invented by Dr. Devi Nambudripad who also wrote a book about it called *Say Goodbye to Illness*. NAET stands for the Nambudripad Allergy Elimination Technique. This is a technique that uses kinesiology and acupressure and/or acupuncture to eliminate allergies. (My doctor uses a variation of the NAET technique that uses only acupressure.) After determining what things you are allergic to, you are put in contact with the allergen during treatment. Then, by opening up the energy pathways of the body (called meridians) using acupuncture (and/or acupressure), NAET retrains the body (and the central nervous system) to "accept" the presence of an allergen instead of viewing it as "foreign". After getting treated for a specific allergen, you no longer have to avoid it. There are no allergy shots or medications involved. In most cases, the allergy is permanently eliminated.

For six months I had treatments to eliminate 32 different allergens. During this time I kept a log of my progress. I was able to notice the connection between certain allergens and certain symptoms. When you are tested for allergies with NAET, it is possible to determine what specific organ against which the allergen causes a reaction and whether you are allergic to it structurally or metabolically. For example, some allergens I was found to be allergic to against my bladder, meaning that when I was exposed to that particular allergen, it would affect my bladder the most. Some things I was allergic to against my thyroid, one was against my lungs, one was against my spleen, and so on. The reason I explain this is because knowing the particular organ(s) that the allergen affected the most, made it quite interesting in terms of the reactions I had after treatments. Basically, I was able to notice the way the allergen had been affecting me.

The connection most pronounced was the connection between the thyroid and the bladder. Every time I was allergic to something against my thyroid, I had bladder symptoms that followed the treatment. When I was treated for allergens against my bladder (which was most of them), then I would feel it in my thyroid. Whenever I was allergic to something structurally, my swelling, muscles and joints would be affected following the treatments. It was all very interesting and I learned that a lot more of my symptoms were allergy related than I had previously thought. With everything new I was learning going through NAET treatments, my opinions about IC kept changing.

I was actually quite surprised to learn not only how many things I was allergic to and in what ways they were effecting me, but also how many things I had been doing on a daily basis thinking they were "good" to do, that were actually causing me more harm than good. For example, I was allergic to corn, and therefore, all corn products. The nutrition drink that I was drinking twice a day had corn syrup in it. So every day my body had to process the "poison" (because that's the way my body saw it; my body saw corn as an allergen or "foreign") from the nutrition drink. The same drink that I thought was helping me was putting even more of a strain on my body. In some respects, it was helping me, but it was also hurting me.

With every treatment I got better and better, even though I did experience a variety of temporary symptoms along the way as my body was re-balancing. It is similar to doing a candida cleanse when you have what are called "die-off" symptoms as the body detoxifies; symptoms that result from the candida dying and trying to leave the body. These symptoms can include things like headaches, intestinal upset, bladder irritation, skin break outs, etc.. With NAET, as allergies are cleared and the body re-balances itself, you will most likely have all kinds of symptoms temporarily. But even with the "side effects", I was still thrilled and excited about my daily progress. There were only two allergens that I had to be re-treated for; that didn't "stick" the first time. Sometimes when the allergy is very strong it takes more than one treatment. I remember wanting to rush through the treatments because I was so excited about getting better. But the faster I went, the harder it was on my body because it had to process all the toxins out after each treatment. So I had to be patient.

Keeping a log not only helped me to notice specific connections between my symptoms and allergies, but also was a great way to keep track of my progress. I remember being so excited the first time I was able to open the dresser drawer to get out a shirt. It was the first time I could do that in over a year. And after being treated for my allergy to vitamin C, my eyes watered for the first time in two years! But looking at my log right now, I also see all the "side effects" and strange pains I went through as I went through these treatments. It's not like it was all a piece of cake, that's for sure. But at the same time, I can still feel the excitement I felt as I read the words I wrote after my seventh treatment...."second day after treatment - FIRST TIME IN OVER THREE YEARS that I'm able to handle the pressure of my hands resting on my bladder/pelvic area as I lie down to sleep!"

Fortunately, by the time this happened with the chemical sensitivities, I had pretty much healed my bladder lining drinking herbal teas. I had worked hard to reduce the swelling, make my muscles stronger and my body less toxic. I don't think there is any way I could have gone through NAET before this point. This is the same way it worked for me

when it came to taking the herbal baths. There was a long time that I couldn't tolerate sitting in a tub of water because of the water pressure. I had to be well enough to do herbal baths, just as I had to be well enough to tolerate the "side effects" of NAET. This is what I mean when I say that you have to judge where you are in the moment with your IC. You are the best judge of your body and only you know what you can tolerate and what you can't. Just because a treatment worked well for one person, does not mean it would be good for you in the situation you're in right now. So even though NAET is something that I would recommend IC patients look into, I also believe that if your bladder is currently in really bad shape, you might want to do other things first so that you can tolerate something like NAET. Or at the very least, go very slowly with the treatments. Keep in mind that anything that processes more toxins out of the body, such as NAET, acupuncture, cleanses, or whatever, will cause some irritation to the bladder. Toxins/poisons have to get out of your body somehow, and one of the ways they do is through the urine. Therefore, doing things to soothe and heal your bladder first, as well as during, these types of treatments is a really good idea.

# Chapter 12

## "It's a combination thing."

Throughout the past few years, almost on a daily basis, Charlie and I would invariably have the same conversation. We were constantly trying to figure out the mysteries of IC, the mysteries behind the different pains and strange unending symptoms. We would consider this and ponder that. Maybe it was what I ate this morning or maybe last night. Maybe it was my stomach or maybe my spleen. Maybe the pain was caused by this or maybe by that. Whatever the specific symptom(s) we were discussing at the moment, the conclusion was always the same. "It's probably a combination thing," we'd say. "Yes...it's most likely a combination thing." When I finally started coming to some conclusions to share with you in this book, I laughed when I realized that what I would be telling you about IC is this...it's a combination thing.

There are many variables that I believe not only cause confusion in trying to understand IC, but are very often present in some form or another in most IC patients. And though they are (or can be) major, bacteria and fungus (yeast) are only two of them. I believe that the cause of IC is a combination of things. *This combination of things produce a continuum of symptoms depending upon the extent to which each of these things are involved.*

It is my belief that IC is even more than a systemic infection. I believe it starts out that way and may even stay that way, but eventually it can involve even more. Some people believe that an initial infection somehow triggers an autoimmune response. Meaning that the body is still fighting infection even after the infection is gone and that the body's own immune system is fighting against itself. And in the absence of apparent infection, IC may appear like an autoimmune disease. I know many IC patients who are convinced that their IC is caused by an autoimmune disease. And there is research to suggest that a protein is present in the urine of IC patients that is not found in healthy controls. The presence of this protein, because it has been found in other autoimmune diseases, seems to suggest that IC could be an autoimmune disease. Some might say that this makes sense because IC is associated with other diseases thought to be autoimmune in nature. But IC is also associated with non-auto-immune diseases as well, such as migraines, IBS, and Fibromyalgia. And who is to say that what is now considered to be an autoimmune disease will not someday be found to be caused by "something". Some people believe that certain autoimmune diseases are really caused by hidden allergies or hidden infections.

## IC and Allergies

Until about a year ago, I didn't understand the relationship between IC and allergies. I mean I knew that allergies were common among IC patients and I knew that I had developed allergies since getting IC (where I had none before), but it wasn't until I was treated with NAET that I learned the magnitude of the relationship. *It is my opinion that once IC is present and the body is all out of balance, allergies can and will develop quickly and worsen with time. It is also interesting to note that long-term use of antibiotics has not only been associated with candida, but has also been associated with the development of allergies.* It is my opinion that IC patients have to be very careful with everything they expose themselves to both internally and externally because allergies can develop very quickly and mysteriously. What never bothered you before your entire life can all of a sudden cause a severe allergic reaction. This happened to me on several occasions.

My experience has taught me that allergies play a major role in IC and in IC related symptoms, certainly more than I had originally thought. They may not be "the" cause, but they most certainly are a factor for most all IC patients. I had no known allergies before I got IC and I developed several (dozens actually) in the past few years since. Allergic reactions can take so many forms and this is something I had never known before. Before I got IC, I thought that allergies meant a stuffy nose, watery eyes, and congestion. You know...like on the commercials. I knew that people allergic to bees could die if they got stung. And that was about all I knew about allergies. My allergies, with the IC, started as sinus-type stuff and congestion (at least as far as I knew). But with time, I developed more and more allergies. Some things I recognized as allergies before I went through NAET treatments, but I also had symptoms that I had absolutely no idea were caused by allergies. This is something I would like to warn you about. You can be allergic to ANYTHING. You can be allergic to vitamins, foods, and things in the environment that you might never imagine. And maybe some of your symptoms can be attributed to allergies and you may not even realize it. I know this was most certainly the case with me.

I assume that you probably have no idea the extent to which allergies are affecting your symptoms. Until your allergies are cleared, you will not really know. I know that NAET may sound like a strange treatment to a lot of people. We are used to taking pills for our symptoms. We are used to blood tests and x-rays and surgery. We are not accustomed to having a non-invasive, painless treatment for IC. (One IC patient I was talking to recently said, "I have to learn that pain does not equal cure". I loved that line. It is so true.) As far as I know, most IC patients deal with their allergies like everybody else, by either trying to avoid the allergen, getting allergy shots, and/or taking antihistamines (if they can tolerate them). I believe NAET is a great alternative to look into for anyone who suffers from allergies.

Some IC patients do notice that when their allergies are worse, their bladder symptoms are worse. Like in the spring, for example, when their seasonal allergies worsen they experience what some IC patients call a "flare". Also, many IC patients recognize that certain foods can cause a "flare", but maybe they don't necessarily relate that to an allergy to a particular food. I know I never did. This is not to say that all reactions to foods for IC patients have to do with allergies. Obviously, there are certain foods that will always irritate a bladder with cuts and/or ulcers, whether you are allergic to them or not.

Some IC patients that recognize allergies as a factor in their IC have determined their allergens by going to an allergist and taking an ELISA/ACT allergy test. Then they try to avoid the allergens to help reduce their symptoms or chances for a "flare". At the very least, this is certainly a good idea to do. You may be aware of your allergies to certain medications or to pollen, for example, but you may not recognize it if you are allergic to calcium or vitamin C, formaldehyde or latex, or even newspaper ink.

Some IC patients are told when they get IC from surgery that maybe they had an allergic reaction to the latex catheter. Actually, this was one of the first things the gynecologist suggested to me following my surgery when he was trying to figure out what was going on. I dismissed it at the time because I knew nothing of latex allergies or what the symptoms might be. And besides, before this surgery, as far as I knew, I wasn't allergic to anything. I didn't realize that I could all of a sudden, for no apparent reason, become allergic to something. Plus, a two-minute conversation with my gynecologist was about as far as it went. It wasn't like he had any suggestions as to what to do about it if a latex allergy was involved or about how to find out if that was actually the case. Besides, I thought, if it was just an allergic reaction, wouldn't the symptoms eventually stop once the allergen was removed? And why would infection accompany it? At the time, I had no idea.

As it turns out, I really was allergic to latex and I do believe it played a part in my IC symptoms. I now know why I was in such agony when they left the catheter in after my cystoscopy. Not only was it because my bladder was irritated and bleeding (which I suppose is bad enough), but also because I had something inserted into my body that I was completely allergic to. The reaction was profound and unforgettable. Yet prior to getting IC, I was not allergic to latex and never had a problem with catheters. We can become allergic to latex (or anything really) almost instantaneously and seemingly spontaneously.

I believe that latex condoms are part of the problem in many cases where an IC patient experiences the onset of symptoms immediately following their first sexual experiences. I also believe a latex allergy is involved when someone gets IC immediately following exposure to a catheter. In both cases, latex is literally inserted into the body. This is not to say that bacteria is not involved, but that the latex catheter (if one were allergic to it) could easily cause a reaction that would compromise the bladder lining making it very susceptible to any bacteria that might be present. *It is also interesting to note that there is current research on resistant bacteria adhering to latex.* Latex is a porous surface and bacteria have been found to stick to it easily.

When we go to the dentist, latex gloves are put into our mouths; when we go to the gynecologist, they wear latex gloves to examine us. If you are allergic to latex and you don't realize it, you will be making yourself more sick every time you are exposed to it. There was an article in the May 1, 1998 edition of Family Practice News magazine called "Latex-Safe Workplace Becoming a Necessity". It explains that 1-6% of the general population is now allergic to latex (which is like millions of people) and that a latex allergy is more common in people with food and environmental allergies. The concern has been raised even higher because a latex allergy is affecting an estimated 12.5% of health care workers in the United States. It is affecting mainstream medicine's own, and is therefore getting some much-needed attention. Thankfully, the necessary changes will also benefit patients as they slowly eliminate latex from the healthcare environment.

Here is one of my many concerns for IC patients. Many IC patients that believe IC is caused by infection are using latex condoms thinking that they are protecting themselves from risk of infection. If they are allergic to latex and don't realize it, it will most certainly be increasing their symptoms. They may be thinking that their symptoms increased from the act of intercourse, but it may have been "a combination thing". I met an IC patient just recently who realized her IC symptoms began right after she started wearing an IUD. In this day and age of sexually transmitted diseases and AIDS, condoms are used more and more often. If you have IC, do yourself a favor and make sure that you are not allergic to latex before using condoms (or catheters for that matter).

Many IC patients believe that they should get a cystoscopy done every once in a while to make sure they don't have cancer or any other problems being masked by their IC symptoms. If they are allergic to latex and don't realize it, the insertion of a catheter during the procedure will make their symptoms worse. I know one IC patient who had no problems with latex catheters for years and then all of a sudden, during a "routine" cystoscopy, she had a huge allergic reaction and her entire vaginal area swelled up three times its normal size. I know countless IC patients who feel much worse after being exposed to catheters during procedures or treatments. Even when initially the catheters/treatments didn't bother them, eventually they say things like "the treatments stopped helping" or "my bladder is much worse since I did the invasive treatments". I've heard both of these comments countless times.

*Repeated exposure to latex promotes the development of a latex allergy.* Combine the fact that IC patients are extra sensitive and known to develop allergies with the fact that IC patients are exposed to latex quite often, and I would say that IC patients who are not allergic to latex initially are certainly ripe to develop this allergy. From diagnosis to treatments, not to mention those getting catheterized in emergency rooms or who self-catheterize at home, latex is all over the place in the world of IC patients.

Many times when an IC patient switches doctors, their new doctor tells them that they want to do another cystoscopy. They want to look inside to see for themselves what is going on. It is my opinion that this will only serve to cause further irritation to the bladder, especially if you are allergic to latex (and even if you're not). Even if you don't believe that a latex allergy is involved in your IC (which I didn't used to either), you can still see why invasive procedures done to your bladder would only serve to further irritate it. If you have already been diagnosed with IC, please give it some extra thought before letting your new doctor put you through yet another cystoscopy so that he can see for himself that you have IC. You might want to ask the doctor what purpose that will serve? Or rather, what purpose will it serve you, the patient? I know IC patients that have had several cystoscopies in the past that didn't bother them, and then all of a sudden, the last one they had caused a tremendous increase in their symptoms. They may have developed a latex allergy since the last time and they didn't know it or their allergic response simply got worse over time, which is typically what allergic responses do.

Here is just one of the problems, in my opinion, with IC treatments today. If a latex allergy is involved with IC patients, the doctors are acting completely unaware of this allergy. In many situations they could be causing more harm to the IC patient by using invasive procedures, which generally include latex gloves and latex catheters.


## IC and the Thyroid

As I mentioned in the last chapter, I definitely noticed a connection between my thyroid and my bladder symptoms when going through NAET. I don't know what the connection is exactly between the thyroid and the bladder, but there sure appears to be one. There are a lot of IC patients who are also diagnosed with hypothyroidism. I know there are some people with IC who have hyperthyroidism, but hypothyroidism seems to be more common. In any case, it seems that

IC patients very often suffer from some type of thyroid problem. Why is this? We know that in the presence of systemic infection, the thyroid is affected. We also know that another cause of thyroid problems is autoimmune disease. *It is interesting to note that nutritional deficiencies and a toxic overload are thought to be the main factors involved in the onset of hypothyroidism.*

When I completed my NAET treatments, I was given a blood test and was found to have hypothyroidism. Several months before I was diagnosed with IC, my old internist had diagnosed me with hypothyroidism. I paid little attention to it because at the time I had zero symptoms of hypothyroidism and I had dozens of symptoms that were still undiagnosed. I was so busy worrying about all the symptoms that I did have, that I put the hypothyroidism on the back burner. I had forgotten all about it until I was told again that I had hypothyroidism. The most noticeable symptom I had that I could directly attribute to my hypothyroidism was pain and swelling in my thyroid. My NAET doctor prescribed some thyroid medication. She prescribed the smallest dosage possible. They were the tiniest little pills I've ever seen. I took one. Of course I had a *huge* reaction to it. Needless to say, I decided not to take the medication and I proceeded to do the same thing I did with everything else. I started reading everything I could about the thyroid and looking for alternative ways to treat the problem. And, as usual, I was trying to understand the possible connections with IC, since when I got IC was when *everything* started for me.

I read both medical articles and alternative medicine articles about hypothyroidism. It was very interesting to me to find out that the symptoms of hypothyroidism very much resembled the list of IC and IC related symptoms. For example, frequent urination, cold hands and feet, inability to sweat and/or night sweats (in other words, abnormal perspiration patterns), very dry skin and hair, environmental and food allergies, premenstrual syndrome and heavy bleeding are all listed as symptoms of hypothyroidism. One article I read about alternative treatments for hypothyroidism actually listed IC as a symptom! Okay I thought, so obviously there was some connection here.

My NAET doctor was open-minded when I suggested that the allergy treatments were the cause of my thyroid getting worse. I believed that all the toxins trying to clear out of my body after the treatments was affecting my thyroid. It certainly was affecting all my other glands. She thought this sounded reasonable. After finding out that it was not urgent that I get on some type of thyroid medication, I told my doctor that I believed I was getting better in every other way and that I was sure I wouldn't have this for the rest of my life either. Just as I knew somewhere inside of me that I wasn't going to have IC forever, I just knew I wouldn't have hypothyroidism forever either. I asked her for some time to try some alternatives, to see if I could get my thyroid better on my own. She was into it. After everything I had been through and how far I had come, I was not about to give up now. I decided, yet again, that I was going to get all the way better.

I learned about a yoga position that you can use to help your thyroid, but I couldn't do it because of the swelling that was still in my upper body. I found other things that I could do instead. I read about how low levels of protein, potassium, and especially magnesium can effect the functioning of the thyroid gland. I changed my diet right away by lowering my carbohydrates and increasing my protein. I read about what foods to avoid and what foods might help my thyroid.

I started using a rebounder (mini-trampoline) to help flush my lymph glands. Initially I could only stand on the rebounder and barely bounce at all with my feet still on the mat. But that was okay. That is called a health bounce and is extremely low impact. Still, I could tell it was helping, just doing that for a minute or so a few times a day. I couldn't believe the difference. Eventually I could jump up a few inches into the air. The rebounding was very helpful and I still do it to this day. It's a very mellow way to flush your lymph system without ingesting anything, which I think is great for IC patients. Rebounding also strengthens all of your internal organs, which is another great thing for IC patients. With the change in diet and the rebounding several times a day, little by little the pain and swelling in my thyroid went down. And once my thyroid and neck felt somewhat better I started swimming again.

At this point I was getting better every day with the swelling all over my body going down gradually, although it was still there. Swimming was helping with the swelling, but still, some remained. As my thyroid improved, my bladder was also improving all the time. At this point I had pretty much healed my bladder all the way and was drinking things like orange juice and coffee with no problem. In general, I was feeling better every day. I had cleared all my allergies and was exercising on a daily basis. I was eating right, meditating every day, getting plenty of rest and had very little stress in my life. My kidneys were better, my thyroid was a lot better, and even my teeth and gums were a little bit better. So why did I still have swelling? Why was my spleen still inflamed? Where were all the toxins coming from? I was missing something and I didn't know what. I prayed for an answer. The very next day I got one.

The next day, I was exposed to cigarette smoke twice, once at a friend's house and once at a restaurant. (I know. Can you believe I could do either one of those things, let alone both in one day?! That's how much better I was doing at this point.) This was the most cigarette smoke I had been exposed to since I had quit smoking and since I had been treated for my subsequent allergy to cigarette smoke. Immediately following exposure to the cigarette smoke, the taste of metal in my mouth came back. This metal taste was familiar because I'd had it from the time I had quit smoking to the time I was treated for my allergy to mercury. As soon as I had been treated for mercury, the metal taste had disappeared. So with the taste of metal in my mouth, I realized that the mercury allergy had returned. I knew I had to go back and get re-treated for the mercury, but I couldn't get an appointment until the following week. Within twenty-four to forty-eight hours all of my symptoms came back. I couldn't believe it! *Everything* came back. The kidney pain, the pain in my spleen, the pain in my thyroid, bladder pain and bladder symptoms of frequency and urgency (if you don't think that freaked me out!), jaw pain, teeth/gum pain, headaches, and IBS symptoms, they all came back. Immediately, I became chemically sensitive again. I couldn't be around perfume, exhaust fumes, or anything with an odor. I was absolutely astounded at the return of *all* of my symptoms. It was so dramatic that it held a major message for me. A message that told me not only to learn more about mercury amalgam fillings, but that there was some major connection here with my IC and my IC related symptoms.

# Chapter 13

❖

# A Missing Piece

Now if someone would have told me a couple of years ago that my IC was in any way related to my teeth, I would have told them that they were crazy. I can't imagine that I would have listened. Actually, I am quite certain that I would not have listened. And I know it sounds crazy, but after the experience I had and after reading about the dangers of mercury amalgam fillings, I now believe that the mercury being released from my dental fillings played a significant role in my IC and my IC related symptoms.

Initially, when I first began to understand the role that allergies play in IC, I thought it was the last piece of the puzzle before I could finish writing this book. I was wrong. And now, as if I'm not talking about enough controversial issues and criticizing the medical community enough, I'm about to bring the dental community in on it as well.

The safety of mercury amalgam fillings is a hot topic among dentists these days. Actually, it has been ever since it first came into use. Dentists in this country are taught that the mercury used in fillings is safe because it is mixed with other metals, and is therefore "sealed" into the filling and not released into the body. We are all told that the mercury in "silver" fillings is not released into our bodies by the mere fact that mercury amalgam is still in use. I think most of us assume that if it were not safe, "they" would not be allowed to use it. When in fact, in many countries, the use of mercury in dentistry has been banned.

# IC and Mercury

If you have silver (sometimes they look black) fillings in your mouth, you have mercury in your mouth. Mercury is the second most toxic metal known in the world. Most people know that mercury is poisonous. This is not news. I remember being taught as a kid that if we ever broke a thermometer we were never to touch the mercury because it was poisonous. Yet, most of us end up with this toxic metal in our mouths. There are numerous research articles pointing to the dangers of mercury amalgam. I could not find one article that said it was safe. Neither could the author of a great book on the subject called *It's All In Your Head - The Link Between Mercury Amalgam and Illness*, written by a dentist, Dr. Hal A. Huggins.

There are several things we know about mercury amalgam fillings; several things that you will come across when you read about them. We know that mercury amalgam fillings consist of 50% mercury, with the remaining 50% being a combination of silver, tin, zinc, and copper. We know that mercury is released into the body when we chew, brush our teeth, and even when we breathe. The older the filling, the greater the corrosion factor. We also know that mercury travels through the body through the blood and lymphatic system, as well as through nerve fibers.

Mercury has been found to accumulate in various organs of the body, including, but not limited to, the brain, the liver, the pituitary gland, the thyroid gland, the kidneys and the female organs. Mercury amalgam fillings have been shown to cause a 50% reduction in kidney filtration function after just two months in the mouth.[2] I found it very interesting that mercury in the body is stored in, filtered through, and directly affects the kidneys. As previously mentioned, there are researchers exploring a toxic substance coming from the kidneys in IC patients. Who knows…maybe mercury is the toxin they are looking for.

Mercury, as you might imagine (being poisonous and all), has also been shown to considerably weaken the immune system. There are numerous studies linking mercury amalgam fillings and endometriosis. I also found this interesting because endometriosis, fibroids, ovarian cysts, and other problems with female organs are very common among IC patients. I also found it interesting that the thyroid gland (and the pituitary gland which directly effects the thyroid's function) is another place where mercury accumulates in the body.

Mercury has also been linked to several autoimmune diseases, such as Multiple Sclerosis, Lupus, and even Parkinson's. It is quite common for researchers to inject mercury into rats when they are trying to produce an autoimmune response for experiments. They use mercury because they often get a 100% success rate in producing the autoimmune response. One reason for this is that mercury binds to proteins. And proteins that have mercury bound to them look like foreign matter to the immune system.

In a 1993 study, the mercury from dental fillings was also shown to increase antibiotic resistance in the bacteria of the gut and mouths of primates.[3] This is yet another interesting connection to IC for those exploring the possibility that IC is caused by a mutated antibiotic resistant organism. *It is also interesting to note that mercury amalgam fillings have been associated with the development of candida AND the development of allergies.*

Curiously, mercury amalgam fillings first came into use in the late 1800's, around the same time that Hunner discovered Hunner's ulcers (or IC). Even more interesting is that during the 1970's the composition of mercury amalgam fillings was changed to include more mercury. It appears to me that in the last 30 years there has been a marked increase in the incidence of IC and IC related illnesses.

As I read about mercury amalgam fillings and noticed all the possible connections with my IC, several things occurred. First and foremost was my decision to have all my mercury fillings replaced with non-metallic composite. Regardless of anything I had read, even the possibility that these fillings could be toxic was enough for me.

Knowing that I had been allergic to mercury, knowing that there was even a possibility that the mercury released from my fillings could be effecting me, and knowing that there is an alternative to mercury amalgam was enough for me. But then I also started remembering things and making connections that I probably would not have been able to make before.

For example, I found it interesting that so many IC patients have sinus problems, jaw pain, TMJ, gum problems, burning tongue or sore tongue, blisters in the mouth or on the throat, earaches and sore throats, swollen glands that don't go away all around the throat, headaches, dry eyes, and dry mouth. Very suspicious for a so-called bladder disease, wouldn't you say? Seems like it's on the wrong end of the body, doesn't it? All of these symptoms can point to mercury poisoning coming from the mouth. The mercury that is released into our mouths gets mixed with our saliva and is constantly being sent into our stomachs and digestive tracts. There are so many IC patients who have an acid stomach, acid reflux, upset stomach with nausea, and symptoms of IBS. So many of us have allergies. So many of us have candida. So many of us seem to have a systemic infection that is not being detected. So many of us have kidney problems and chemical sensitivities. All of these things can point to mercury poisoning.

Of course, not all IC patients will necessarily have problems with their mercury fillings. In fact, not all IC patients will even HAVE mercury amalgam fillings (crowns or root canals). But if you do have mercury in your mouth and you have IC, I would certainly consider it a possibility that they are part of the problem, or should I say, contributing to the problem.

There are clearly people out there who have mercury amalgam fillings in their mouths and have no obvious adverse reactions, where other people are more sensitive. (Gee…I wonder what category IC patients fit in. Just kidding.) There are a few different factors that might effect why some people are bothered more than others by their mercury fillings. At first it was believed that the more mercury excreted through

114

the urine of test patients meant that they were the most toxic. And then they discovered that those who excrete higher levels of mercury in their urine might not have as much of a problem with mercury as someone who has lower levels. This is what they call mercury retention. This is when the body is not processing the mercury out and more is being stored in the body. The more mercury being stored in the body, the greater the chance it will cause health problems. Another factor could be the acid/alkaline balance in the mouth. Some have pointed to the electrical charge between the different metals in the mouth to be a cause. Another could be the actual number of mercury amalgam fillings. Of course, being allergic to mercury is certainly a significant factor in whether or not your fillings will affect your health. Also, it has been noticed that crowns and root canals are the worst because the mercury is either closer to the gums (being underneath the crown) or actually inserted down into the root, as in the case of a root canal.

Some people who suspect their mercury fillings are related to their health problems have their fillings removed. Some notice an improvement in their health problems, while others do not. Even if you've had your mercury fillings removed, mercury can *still* be stored in your organs and still be affecting your health. Especially if you were prone to mercury retention and it wasn't getting flushed out of your body properly to begin with. So it is very important to cleanse the mercury out of the body during and/or after getting your fillings removed.

As I began to have my fillings replaced and became more resolved in the fact that there was some kind of connection here with my symptoms, I happened to run across an old e-mail from a couple years ago. It was from my friend Jill who usually copies what I write into her e-mail and then writes her reply underneath. So I was able to see what I had written her over two years ago, shortly after Charlie and I had returned home from our wedding. I had told her about how everything was going just fine until I went to the dentist, had a couple of fillings replaced and then got a huge kidney infection the very next day. I had no idea! I didn't remember that at all. I thought I had just gotten too worn out from traveling and the wedding and everything. When I saw that e-mail I couldn't believe my eyes! I had actually had two large fillings replaced with "silver" (because what did I know at the time) right before my kidneys got really bad. Very interesting, I thought.

With each filling that I had replaced, I saw improvements in my symptoms. The right side of my sinuses began to drain for the first time in three years. The swollen glands under my arms and all around my neck began to go down…finally! My thyroid got better and the moisture returned to my eyes and mouth. My skin broke out all over, especially my chest and arms, as the mercury left my body. And just as with NAET and the candida cleanse, there were toxins/poisons to process and flush out of my body as I had each tooth done. My swelling began to go down all over my body. As my swelling went down, my strength and flexibility started coming back. My chemical sensitivities also got better with each filling I had replaced. I started being able to tolerate being around perfume, exhaust fumes, and cigarette smoke. And I also noticed a connection with my Vulvodynia symptoms.

Many IC patients, myself included, consider Vulvodynia to be "IC on the outside". It is the same irritation on external tissues as we have within the urethra and bladder. For many of us our IC symptoms and Vulvodynia symptoms coincide. When the IC flares, so does the Vulvodynia. Many of us have a clear mysterious discharge and no one really knows what it is. Some people may feel it as moisture and not realize it is discharge because it is clear. Some have it cultured and often nothing is found. Just as some IC patients believe that the onset of their symptoms began after using antibiotics, so do many Vulvodynia patients. Yet when tested, yeast does not always show on the culture. I would suggest that maybe what they should be looking for is mercury.

I know my Vulvodynia symptoms were directly related to my IC. And the clear mysterious discharge, for me, was directly related to my teeth. As I was getting my fillings replaced, it became very obvious to me as this symptom returned temporarily. The serious increase in discharge, as well as the return of the Vulvodynia symptoms, was directly related to the mercury being released out of my body. This made a lot of sense to me as mercury is often stored in the female organs. This release also occurred when I was cleared of my mercury allergy with NAET. And when it happened again with each filling I had replaced, it made me more certain than ever that the mercury was related. It is no wonder that nothing is usually found in the cultures.

It is not that I believe that mercury amalgam fillings caused my IC. But I do believe they played a significant role in many of my symptoms. I believe that having IC made me much more susceptible to developing allergies and having the mercury in my fillings effect me so much, though it could have just as easily been the other way around. If I knew then what I know now, I would have had my fillings replaced much earlier on.

Almost the entire time I had IC, I treated myself as if I had a systemic infection; as if I were completely toxic and full of poison/acid in my system. This is what IC felt like to me. This is what my symptoms were pointing to. This approach was a major factor in how I got well. Even after fighting the infection and soothing my insides, I still had to get to the bottom of all the other sources of toxins/poisons in my system, whether they be from smoking, allergens, or mercury. I also found it necessary to eliminate all the allergies that had developed since I got IC by re-balancing my body with the NAET treatments. And lastly, I found it absolutely necessary to remove my mercury amalgam fillings.

# Chapter 14

◆

# Healing Pains and Healing Joys

Aside from the fact that we are all different when it comes to our symptoms and our responses to treatments, one thing that was very difficult for me as I was trying to get better was that I was the only IC patient that I knew of trying or doing the particular things I did to get well. For example, at the time I was doing the anti-candida program, I didn't know any other IC patients trying colloidal silver or doing an anti-candida program. Though most likely there had been others before me, at the time, there wasn't anyone on line that I knew of to ask questions. And when I first began drinking Marshmallow Root tea or when I was going through NAET treatments, no other IC patients that I knew had ever heard of either. Even when I was taking herbal baths or having my fillings replaced, I didn't know a single IC patient who I could ask if what I was going through was "normal". So all of these things I did were "new" to me and generally were not accepted as "normal" treatments for IC. I really had to learn to trust myself, because I'll tell you this...healing is NOT pain free.

There are decisions to make, dosages to adjust, symptoms to deal with, and fear to contend with. Just as muscles and broken bones hurt as they heal, so do internal organs. Staying in touch with my body and noticing how I was feeling was very important. Keeping track of what I was doing was also important so that I could tell if it was helping or hurting. Sometimes, even though it felt as if what I was doing was hurting me physically, I would still know that it was a good thing. There is discomfort as your body heals and there are various symptoms that occur whenever you detoxify your body.

There were times when my swelling was going down that it was extremely painful in my muscles and joints, but I knew my swelling was going down, so I didn't mind as much. There were times when my kidneys were sore or my spleen hurt, but I knew I was passing toxins/poisons out of my system, so I tried not to worry about it. There were times when my bladder pain and symptoms returned temporarily as I was cleansing out the toxins and poisons, but I knew I was detoxifying my body, so I wasn't too worried. Okay...that one's not true. Actually, it was scary every time the bladder pain returned, but I tried really hard not to be scared.

Healing was not always easy. It took a long time and a lot of work to get to this point. There was a lot I had to give up temporarily, like coffee and sodas, chocolate and sex. And some things I had to give up permanently, like smoking cigarettes and certain people in my life. And there were some new things that I had to learn to do that I had never done before, like pay attention to my diet and meditate. As I was getting better, I also had to learn to be out in the world again. It had been over a year since I had driven a car and a few years since I had gone out to dinner with other people, or anywhere else for that matter. It was like I had to learn how to talk to people all over again. Sure I was talking to IC patients all the time, but it wasn't the same thing as making dinner conversation with people Charlie works with, for example. I remember joking around with some of my IC friends about how we were afraid that we would become agoraphobic (afraid to leave the house) after being housebound with IC for so long. And though it was a joke, there was still some truth to it.

As I mentioned earlier, it took a lot of things for me to get better from IC. Between the antibiotics, anti-candida program, herbs and acupressure, eliminating allergies with NAET, and removing my mercury amalgam fillings, I went through a lot of different phases in my symptoms and treatment. People often ask me what helped me the most and what would I do differently. These are tough questions to answer, but I'll do my best because I know many people will wonder this very thing. What helped me the most? 1) Staying away from invasive procedures was very important in allowing my bladder a chance to heal. Each cystoscopy and examination I had caused more pain and damage to my bladder. I am forever grateful to have found other IC patients to talk to so that I was able to avoid the painful, invasive procedures that were being recommended to me by the doctor. 2) Staying away from synthetic medications, as much as possible, I feel was also very important. I'm all for pain medication and not being in pain, but avoiding other synthetic medications, I believe, gave my body and bladder a much better chance to heal. I still believe that other medications only add more chemicals to an IC patient's already toxic body. 3) Healing my bladder lining (and my kidneys) with marshmallow root tea (and comfrey leaf tea). 4) Boosting my immune system with herbs and nutrition. 5) Fighting infections with natural things instead of synthetic antibiotics. 6) Eliminating my allergies with NAET. 7) Replacing my mercury amalgam fillings. 8) Meditation, relaxation, and stress reduction also helped my immune system get stronger and my body to heal. 9) And lastly, the belief that I would get well.

What would I do different? 1) I would still take antibiotics first if my bladder was bleeding like it was, but I probably wouldn't have stayed on them for as long as I did (4 months). I would have switched over to natural antibiotics a lot sooner. 2) I would have taken more acidophilus while I was on antibiotics. 3) I would have waited to quit smoking until I was already undergoing NAET treatments. 4) I would have replaced my mercury amalgam fillings MUCH sooner. 5) I would have been nicer to myself.

At the time of this writing, I have one more filling left to be replaced. I've already had twelve done, along with a crown. I've gotten better and better with each filling I've had replaced. Actually, there has been a phenomenal improvement in all of my symptoms. One thing that I want you to know is that everything goes back to normal when you get better. Vaginal moisture, the strength of your pelvic floor muscles, your sex drive, the force of your urine stream; it all goes back to normal. Other IC patients always ask me whether I can have sex without pain, whether I can eat and drink what I want, whether I am free of bladder pain and symptoms. The answer is yes to all of these.

Charlie and I celebrated every small step along the way. If I was able to go to the grocery store with him, we would be thrilled. If I made it on a car ride without having to stop every five minutes, we were hopeful. If I was able to open the refrigerator door and take out the half-gallon milk container, we were jumping for joy at my progress. To this day I am overjoyed that I can flush the toilet with one hand (there was at least a month with the fibromyalgia where I couldn't even flush using both hands) and walk down the steps barely holding onto the railing. I'm always turning around at the bottom of the steps yelling to Charlie, "Did you see that?! Did you see that?!" I celebrate every time I take a shower because I'm no longer in agony when the water hits my body. I appreciate every little thing. I can't even help it.

I can't guarantee you how I'm doing at the time you're reading this, but hopefully I am completely back to "normal", as I am almost there now. There was a long time when I was first sick that I wasn't making any improvements. At that time, each day felt the same, if not worse, than the day before. Once I got some understanding of what was going on inside my body and then started treating it accordingly, I started getting better. Because I had such a dramatic onset to my IC, it was easier for me to see that it was all one thing. I know it is much more difficult when your symptoms develop over time. I know that many IC patients feel like their bodies are falling apart; that they are just gigantically unlucky and that for some unknown reason they have developed several incurable chronic illnesses. Over time they go to different specialists and get multiple diagnoses and then they think they have several different diseases. It is my impression that they are very often related.

I also can't guarantee you that the way I did things will be the way that will work for you, but I can guarantee you that there **is** hope for you to get better. As I said earlier, we are all at a different place with our IC and we all have a slightly different path. But I believe that if you address your whole body, rather than just your bladder, you will have the best chance. It has been my experience that bacteria, candida, allergies, the thyroid, and mercury amalgam fillings can all be factors contributing to the overall IC experience. It is my opinion that these factors are somehow all connected and that individually we experience some, or all of them, to a different degree. As I've mentioned before, I believe IC patients have toxic bodies, everyone to a different degree. Not only that, but we are not all becoming toxic for the same exact reasons. There are many things that cause a toxic environment within the body. And a toxic environment within the body is what allows IC to thrive. To make things more confusing, we all have different physical weaknesses and we all develop different allergies. We can even have different allergic reactions to the exact same allergen. (For example, maybe I am allergic to Percocet and when I take it I get severe stomach pains and feel like I overdosed. And maybe you are also allergic to Percocet, but it makes you break out in hives.) I believe these are reasons why everyone's symptoms seem to be different, why our reactions to treatments and medications are not always the same, and why what works for one of us, doesn't necessarily work for another. I believe we have to look at our own individual situation in order to determine what needs to be addressed and how. If our doctor is not looking at our symptoms "all together", then I think we need to be. We need to take responsibility for researching our own treatments and deciding what is best for our own bodies.

There are some days when you will feel as if you have a handle on the situation and other days when you will feel panic stricken and have no idea whether you're doing the right thing; no idea what to do next. I want to be able to tell you that it will be easy. I want to be able to tell you that there is a quick fix for IC and that you'll be better soon if you just follow this treatment or take this pill. I know that's what you want. Hell...I know that's what I wanted. I wish I could tell you that if you just go to Dr. So and So that he/she could cure you in a minute. But instead I tell you this. No one else can or will get you better from IC. Only you can get yourself well. There is no magic cure and there is no "IC expert". We have to be our own IC expert. Pray for a cure, yes, but don't just sit back and wait. Go to the doctor, yes, but don't obey him/her without question or research on your part. Mainstream medicine has not yet offered us a cure, and I for one was not willing to wait for them to figure it out. Just because "they" say IC is incurable, doesn't mean that it is. It just means that "they" haven't figured it out yet. For every disease "they" say is incurable, there is someone out there who has "cured" themselves. Now you have met one.

*Alternative ways...*

# Chapter 15

◆

# Alternative Healers and Therapies

Psychic healers and medical intuitives are certainly not for everyone. But in moments of desperation and in trying to figure out some direction to take, I have consulted a few reputable healers with the ability to see into the body. This is not to say that the basis for my opinions about IC are completely based on their insights, but it did provide some confirmation to what I was surmising from the literature, my experience, and the experiences of other IC patients.

Before I was diagnosed with IC, I went to a psychic healer/medical intuitive to get her perspective on what was going on inside my body. I had met her prior to getting sick and remembered that her specialty was health. The doctors couldn't figure out what was wrong with me, so I thought this might offer me some insight. If I disagreed, I knew I didn't have to listen to or act on what she told me. And I thought maybe this might give me some direction or some ideas of things to look into. At this point, I was still searching through those giant medical books trying to figure out what was wrong with me.

As soon as I walked through the door, the first thing that Cynthia said to me was "Oh my God! There's poison all over your body! There's poison all over your body!" She wanted to know what "they" did to me and had me sit down right away. She said I had no business being out and about. My aura looked greenish-brown. She said I "looked" awful. Like most people, Cynthia had never heard of IC. Actually, she didn't mention my bladder at all during this first visit. What she described was poison in my blood. She recognized that I had candida, but said this was not all that was going on. She mentioned that she didn't like my doctor. Being as skeptical as I had always been, I didn't listen to much of what she told me on that first visit. It took me over a year before I looked at candida in relation to IC. And that was only because I ended up taking antibiotics. It also took several months before I learned that the doctor I liked, the one who saved my life when I had internal bleeding, was the same doctor who covered up for his associate and did not do a surgical report for my surgery. And most importantly, it took a long time before I realized what it meant when Cynthia said "there's poison all over your body!".

Since then, Cynthia and I have become friends and she has helped me on several occasions to figure out what was going on inside my body so that I could determine what to do next. And even though I didn't always listen to her, there were many times where later she would prove to have been right. There were also times she was not quite as accurate. No psychic can be accurate 100% of the time. I would listen to her and then decide whether or not I agreed. I would research everything and then follow my gut instincts. So sometimes I listened and other times I didn't. I looked at it as one more alternative when I was looking for insight.

A medical intuitive can have a range of abilities. From seeing into the body to being able to "read" the energy or aura around a person, to getting psychic messages through clairvoyance regarding illness within the body. Some can do all of these things. This is true for psychic healers as well. They might use Reiki (or the laying on of hands), psychic surgery, or long distance healing. Some use crystal healing, toning, or contact healing. Some may use all of these techniques depending on how they are guided. There are so many healing methods and so many abilities. The healers I spoke to and worked with directly had a variety of abilities. My friend Cynthia had them all. She is what they call a mystic.

It is interesting to note that healers from different parts of the country, unbeknownst to each other, all reported basically the same "vision" of IC. I thought it was important to share what they "saw" as some might be interested in their insights.

Psychic healers/medical intuitives see IC as a viral bacteria. Some say it is more like a virus than a bacteria. But basically they all say that it is both in one microscopic organism that cannot be detected through "normal" routine cultures. It is a mutated, antibiotic resistant bacteria with a translucent cell wall. (Dr. Durier seems to have come the closest with his cell wall deficient bacteria theory.) IC, they believe, is a systemic infection. The bacteria gets into the bloodstream in various ways and then flows throughout the body and manifests in the weakest organs. Some bacteria are gram positive and some are gram negative. The IC bacteria is gram negative according to Cynthia. Some bacteria release acid and others do not. The IC bacteria releases acid. IC flows through the digestive system and works its way out through the urinary tract. And when it does, it's a high acid, a burning poison, which eats away at the layers of skin, or rather, mucous membranes. IC attacks the bladder first and then spreads microscopically throughout the body. According to the psychic healers I worked with, IC travels in the blood and other bodily fluids (including spinal fluid). It has been likened to boric acid, a poison in the body.

There does appear to be a viral component to IC. It very often appears to lie dormant in the body and then comes back. I know many of us have experienced a similar phenomenon. When we get the flu or some other virus, it seems to put our IC into temporary remission, only to return when the flu disappears. A similar thing occurs during pregnancy for some people. It's as if the IC goes into remission to protect the baby and then returns when the baby is born.

Aside from their view of IC, there are also several other things I learned from going to healers. The most important thing I learned was that *we are the ones who heal ourselves*. I learned not to put too much faith into any type of healer, whether a psychic healer or medical doctor. I have found that it is better to believe in your own ability to heal yourself (because we all do have this ability), rather than believing that another person is going to heal you. Also, just as you often can't reach your doctor on the phone, the same can be true with psychic healers. They may not always be available to you when you need them. Going to psychic healers also helped me learn to listen to my body more and often confirmed my feelings and suspicions. *Most importantly, I learned not to give over "control" to any other healer but myself.*

If you are considering going to a psychic healer/medical intuitive, know that a true healer will not take money for healings. They might take money for readings, but not for healings. Know that it should not cost you a lot of money for this type of help. Remember to do only what feels comfortable to you. A healer should make you feel comfortable, not afraid. Most importantly, they should empower you, not take your power. In other words, they should be helping you to take control of your own health situation versus them taking control of it for you. They should be telling you that *you are the one who heals yourself.* If they tell you that they are the one who is healing you, find somebody else.

Obviously, there are several types of alternative healers besides psychic healer/medical intuitives. Some of them have a medical background and others do not. For example, a holistic doctor is a doctor who looks at the whole body when treating disease. They might use homeopathic remedies, vitamins, and herbs or even synthetic medications in treating patients. Holistic simply means looking at the whole body; it does not determine what types of treatments the doctor uses. A naturopath is someone who uses natural treatments. Again, they can be any variety of natural treatments. An herbologist is someone who specializes in herbs and usually vitamins too. An osteopath is a medical doctor trained in the manipulation of bones similar to a chiropractor. All of these, including acupuncturists and massage therapists, are considered alternative healers.

There are alternative therapies that are wonderful for certain things, but I still would not advise them for IC patients. Certain therapies can be too strong for someone with IC. We are very sensitive and have to be more careful than many of these "healers" will understand. *You have to warn them about this and you may have to be assertive and tell them no*. Obviously, it's not that they will be trying to hurt you. It just may happen because of their lack of understanding of IC. This is no different, in my opinion, than dealing with medical doctors.

I understand that many of you reading this may be afraid to go out and try alternative treatments. Maybe you just don't know where to begin. Maybe you are like I was and you don't know much about alternative treatments. I will try to help by providing some examples of what I did and try to warn you of some things to be careful of. Please, though, whatever it is that catches your interest, read more about it elsewhere. I assure you that I am not an expert on any of these methods.

Things to be careful of...

Kinesiology is a form of muscle response testing. It is based on the premise that there is an important interrelationship between various muscle groups and specific body systems and that the strength of the muscle, when tested, displays a reflection of the state of its related organ/tissues. It is often used as a diagnostic tool and to help determine what vitamins and herbs (and in what quantities) may be appropriate. Just because you are muscle tested by a kinesiologist and are told that your body "needs" a specific product or vitamin/herb, does not mean that your bladder or body can tolerate it. You may *still* have a reaction. Please keep this in mind if you go to an alternative practitioner who tells you to take a whole list of vitamins and herbs. If you end up buying all sorts of vitamins and herbs and believe that they are the right things for you to take, do yourself a giant favor and try one at a time...with the smallest dose possible.

Acupuncture, in my opinion, is too strong for many IC patients. Though if you have mild symptoms, I would consider trying it. It is an excellent way to re-balance the body and has been used for centuries to do so. If you think it may be too strong for you and you feel very toxic or infected, I would attempt to cleanse out some of the poisons first in other more gentle ways and then later maybe you can try acupuncture if you are so inclined.

Though I'm quite sure that homeopathic medicine is wonderful for certain illnesses, I strongly believe that it is not for IC patients. The basis for homeopathic medicine is to give the body some of what it is already fighting in order to boost the immune system into fighting it harder. I believe IC patients, in general, are too toxic and often too sick for this type of medicine. Homeopathic remedies are something that IC patients should be extremely careful with and would be best to avoid. Personally, I had terrible experiences with homeopathic medicine, which I tried on two different occasions in extremely low doses. If you are inclined to try a homeopathic remedy, please be very careful and take only one drop in a glass of water the first time you take it. This way, if your body reacts poorly, you won't have ingested more than a drop. Even if the bottle or a doctor tells you to take four drops in water (or whatever the instructions), *still* start out by only taking one drop in water. And even then you might want to drink only a few sips of the water. This is how strong homeopathy is for IC patients. Even that one drop in a glass of water may cause a severe negative reaction in your body. Besides, you can always increase your dosage later if you find that your body can handle it.

Intrinsically, there is nothing wrong with Chinese herbs, of course. But Chinese herbs are typically very strong and personally, I would avoid these also if you have IC. I know that there is a doctor in Philadelphia that uses a combination of Chinese herbs in a tea made especially for IC patients. If you try them and can tolerate them, then great, but many of you may not be able to tolerate them. Don't let this discourage you from taking other herbs. Just steer clear of anything harsh and go for the soothing, more gentle herbs.

The same caution should be applied to cleanses (i.e., products used to cleanse toxins out of the body). There are tons of different types of cleanses on the market. Please be *very* careful with cleanses. Though I do believe it is important for IC patients to cleanse the toxins/poisons out of their bodies, I would advise you to be really, really careful *how* you do it. For example, you might see some de-tox herbal combination teas or other herbal cleanses at the health food store. These are most likely *way* too strong. Almost any cleansing product you will find at the health food store will most likely be way too strong. But if you find a really mild one you want to try, I would just start out with the absolute smallest dosage possible. You might hear of using lemon juice as a cleanse, garlic or cayenne pepper as a treatment for infection. Do yourself a big favor and stay FAR away from those. They will most likely cause a lot of pain for IC patients. A lot of pain. I would also advise staying away from cranberry juice and Uva Ursi (which is an herb often recommended for urinary tract infections). Both are good for the urinary tract/bladder for normally healthy people, but are typically *way* too strong for IC patients and can really cause a lot of irritation making the pain, and you, much worse. Use common sense in terms of what will burn an already irritated, inflamed, and/or bleeding bladder.

# Chapter 16

———◆———

# Alternatives You Can Try
# At Home

There are so many things you can try...never think you don't have any options. As promised, these are all things that I did to get better, starting with the most simple and obvious. These are not all literally "alternative" things, but they are all things that your medical doctor will probably not be discussing with you, so I have included them here.

Maybe you are like me and would not have considered treatments such as these to be valid or even an option prior to getting IC. But maybe with the choices that are available to IC patients today, you are willing to consider them. Or if you are like me and would prefer to try as many non-invasive treatments first, then you might also want to consider them. And lastly, if you are looking for options because you've already tried everything that's currently being offered by the medical community, then at least you know there are choices.

**Good nutrition** is so important. Unlike adherence to the IC diet, good nutrition often goes unmentioned. It is my opinion that IC bodies are not absorbing nutrition. Most often, the stomach and digestive tract is affected by IC, just like the urinary tract. It doesn't matter whether you see it as candida or irritable bowel syndrome. Some IC patients have been diagnosed with colitis or diverticulitis. Some have acid reflux or stomach ulcers. No matter what you call it, most IC patients know that their digestive systems are effected somehow. We need to help our bodies to get extra nutrition because the food we are eating is not necessarily going to be enough to provide the necessary nutrients for our bodies to heal.

Many IC patients find it difficult to eat much of anything. Between the IC diet, the anti-candida diet and the low oxalate diet, it can be very confusing and frustrating just trying to find something to eat. And trying to determine and avoid foods that bother you, while still getting enough nutrition at the same time, is definitely not easy. But it's important to at least try to make certain you are getting the nutrition you need to heal.

Eating as many fresh, whole foods as possible (that your bladder can tolerate of course) is very important. Here are some examples of what I did. I used to eat fresh parsley (which is great for the bladder and urinary tract), alfalfa sprouts, sliced carrots, and baby spinach salads. Celery (or celery seed) is also good for the bladder and urinary tract. I used to drink an herbal nutrition drink that helped me rebuild my body after I had lost over twenty pounds when I was first sick. Later, when my bladder was a lot better, I switched to a homemade nutrition drink that Charlie invented for me. It included a banana, a chocolate Ensure (I know that chocolate is an IC no-no, but by this time I had healed my bladder enough to tolerate it.), a couple tablespoons of strawberry liquid acidophilus, three or four heaping tablespoons of plain low-fat yogurt with acidophilus, a protein (amino acid) pill crunched up, and a few drops of liquid concentrated minerals. It tasted like a milkshake, which is what got me to drink it. There were times I drank it twice a day when I felt I wasn't getting enough nutrition from the food I was eating. Nutrition drinks are also great because you don't have to get as full, which as you know can often cause more pressure, bloating and pain. There are several kinds of nutrition drinks at the health food store. Just find one that you can tolerate and one that you like enough that you can drink it everyday (or when you need to). Once my bladder lining was healed, Charlie and I got a juicer and started juicing fruits and vegetables. But please don't try that until your bladder is healed or it will most likely cause some serious pain.

***Flush your body every day with lots of distilled water***. When I first got sick I had no idea the importance of drinking a lot of water. I was already going to the bathroom every five-ten minutes and the last thing I thought I needed was more liquid. Plus, I was afraid of filling my bladder at all because it was so incredibly painful. My bladder was so raw that I couldn't stand to have even a few drops of urine in it, let alone a whole glass of water! I was also afraid because so often I couldn't even go and then the more full my bladder became, the more pain, nausea, and panic I felt. I didn't know back then that my urine was so toxic. I didn't realize that if I drank more water it would dilute the urine and therefore hurt less. No one had explained to me WHY I couldn't go when my bladder was so full. I didn't realize then that the bladder gets distended when it's full and if it has cuts and/or ulcers that are getting irritated, the bladder spasms. So diluting the urine with lots of water is also helpful in cutting down on the bladder spasms. Back then I also didn't realize the importance of flushing my body with water every day for not only my bladder, but for the rest of me as well. Again, because I didn't realize that it was a great way to gently flush the toxins out of my body.

Water is very healing. After all, our bodies are made up of mostly water and we need water to survive. *Water for the IC patient is essential.* Unfortunately I've heard on several occasions of urologists telling IC patients to cut down on their fluid intake "if you are going to the bathroom so much...don't drink so much", they tell them. This is some really bad advice. I know IC patients who get dehydrated quite often and end up in the hospital because they are avoiding drinking water. They aren't doing it "on purpose", they are doing it for the same reasons I mentioned above that I was afraid to drink too much water.

When it comes to water, distilled is often considered better than spring water. This is because water advertised as distilled has to be distilled, but spring water can be anything. But please keep in mind that distilled water is also void of many of the minerals that non-distilled water would contain. So if you are drinking distilled water, it's a good idea to get minerals from other sources. I do know several people who found a specific spring water they liked and then stuck to that. Whatever you do, do not drink tap water.

Learning and using **acupressure points** at home is easy. Acupressure is a great way to rebalance the body. It is based on the same premise as acupuncture, but with acupressure there are no needles. You simply press on the points with your fingers instead, making it a simple and painless way to help your body repair itself without ingesting anything. Get one or two books. They generally have pictures and show you what pressure points coincide with what organs. Believe me, you don't have to be a genius to press on acupressure points, although it is important not to overdo it. When I first got my acupressure books, I would experiment learning the pressure points, pressing on all these different points to see which ones hurt, and I ended up making myself get poison rushes and feel really sick. This is similar to those who have tried acupuncture and found it to be way too strong. So be careful when you start experimenting. But other than that, you can't really hurt yourself doing acupressure as far as I know. If points don't hurt, you don't need to use them. Your body will tell you what it needs. And if you start to feel crummy, stop pressing. It's pretty simple to be able to control the intensity. I used acupressure points to help clear congestion, to flush excess water from my body, to flush my lymph system, and to relieve pain.

**Reflexology** is based on the premise that there are areas on the feet and hands that correspond to all body parts. Reflexology helps nature to normalize body functions by releasing tension build-up from toxins in various parts of the body. Reflexology is also very easy to learn to do at home. You can get a book or even just a chart. You can buy a reflexology chart for a little over a dollar and there are many books out there on reflexology. I think that once you start using this, you will be astounded how the painful areas on your feet completely coincide with what is hurting on your body. Don't overdo the foot massages either. The more sick you are, the more your feet will hurt to be touched. When I was really sick, Charlie would barely touch my feet and I would be in tears. If my bladder wasn't working due to spasms, Charlie would give me a foot massage and often it would help me be able to go. Whether it was helping to "flush" my body or whether it was just helping me to relax from the pain, I'm not sure, but most likely it was a combination thing. Always drink a lot of water following a foot massage. Actually, you should drink a lot of water after doing anything that helps flush toxins out of your body.

**Massage** is also very helpful. Even light massage will help move the lymph system and help to release toxins from the muscles. It is also excellent for stress reduction, relaxation, and helps pain in the muscles and joints typically associated with fibromyalgia and IC. If you can't afford to or are not well enough to go to a massage therapist, try bribing someone who loves you. I used to tell Charlie that I'd give him a million dollars for a foot massage. (Be careful though, I currently owe him over 12 billion dollars.) Again, always drink a lot of water following any type of massage to help flush the toxins from your body.

**Herbs** are used to help the body heal itself. This is where herbs are different from medications. In general, herbs aid in the body's natural healing versus covering up symptoms like synthetic medications often do. There are herbs to boost the immune system, to help soothe organs, to clear congestion, to soothe aching muscles, or to fight infection.

Herbs can be taken in many forms. You can drink herbs in a tea, take herbs in a tincture (i.e., a concentrated liquid form), or take them in capsule form. After determining which herb you are going to take and why, you still have to determine *how* you are going to take it and how much. This is what people find most difficult. The directions on the bottle are often vague and you're never sure if they apply to you or your particular situation. My rule of thumb on how much to take is as follows. *Always start out with the smallest dosage possible.* Don't follow the directions on the side of the bottle. These amounts are for "normal" people, not IC patients. Make sure you are able to determine your reaction to the particular herb you are trying. Therefore, do not try more than one herb at a time. Try not to change anything else the day you try the new herb. For example, don't eat food that you normally never eat or go somewhere new where you might be exposed to something you aren't normally exposed to. This way you can tell that you are reacting to what you have taken and not something else.

When it comes to deciding what form of the herb to take, I always kept the following in mind. An herbal tincture is best absorbed in the blood. Usually you take a few drops under the tongue, a place known to absorb quickly into the blood stream. (They do make non-alcohol tinctures and these are definitely what I would recommend for IC patients.) Herbal capsules are best absorbed through the digestive system as they are swallowed and then dissolved in the stomach. And teas are best absorbed throughout all the tissues.

I believe herbal teas are wonderful for IC patients for many reasons. You can make them as weak as you want and only have a few sips at a time. Therefore, you can take the herb, but in a very low dose. And this is very often all you will be able to tolerate. I didn't realize when I first started using herbs that it was okay to take such a small dose. You would think that it wouldn't do much of anything. But this is not true. Very often, for IC patients, it is enough. Many IC patients have tried various herbs and find that they have a strong reaction to them. It could be that they were taking too strong a dose or it could be that they were allergic to them. That's why trying herbs in a tea is so great. You can take a couple sips, instead of a whole capsule, to make sure you can tolerate them first. If you are trying an herb in capsule form, you can even open the capsule and only take part of it the first time.

I believe it is best to *stick with single herbs*. If you are buying herbal tea, I wouldn't buy it in the tea bags. Very often, tea bags have many different herbs in them, with some that you can tolerate and maybe others that you can't. IC patients are better off taking single herbs and buying them in bulk form. This way you can take them one at a time and it will be easier to determine whether you can tolerate them and/or how they are effecting you. I think you will find that there are more herbs that you are able to tolerate this way as well.

How to buy herbs - For the most part, I buy my herbs from an herb farm. They are fresh and inexpensive. I find this to be the best way to buy herbs in bulk for tea. I buy herbal capsules, tinctures, and essential oils at the health food store. I always used non-alcohol tinctures for my IC. You will usually have to go to a mom and pop type health food store to find what you're looking for. If they don't have what you're looking for, they are usually able to order it for you. These days there are about a million different companies that sell vitamins and herbal products. You really have to do some research and decide what company you like and trust. I found a couple that I liked and generally stuck with them.

Specifically the herbs that I used…

At various times and for various reasons I took the following herbs to help heal my bladder and my body from IC. I have listed them in order of significance to my healing.

The number one herb that I have been telling IC patients about the past couple of years is Marshmallow Root. It is the herb, I believe, that contributed the most to healing my bladder lining. Though I did take the non-alcohol Marshmallow Root tincture for my kidneys and the capsules for my intestines, I drank it in a tea most often. Marshmallow Root has been called the aloe vera for internal organs. It is very soothing and healing to the tissues of the kidneys, urinary tract, and bladder.

Marshmallow Root does not build up over time. It is not like bladder coating drugs that take time to build up and eventually coat the bladder wall. Rather, it is soothing to the tissues of the bladder and will help to heal (or rebuild) the bladder lining, as opposed to temporarily coating it. I think it is better than bladder coating drugs for several reasons. First and foremost because it is non-toxic and it doesn't have any side effects. (Actually, I should say that it *shouldn't* have any side effects. In other words, if you do experience side effects from Marshmallow Root, then you are probably allergic to it.) Secondly, it does not take months to work. Thirdly, you don't have to take it the rest of your life. And lastly, it doesn't cost a small fortune. Actually, you can get a big bag of Marshmallow Root for just a couple dollars. However mild or severe your bladder symptoms, Marshmallow Root tea is something I would strongly recommend.

Marshmallow Root is often used as an anti-irritant and anti-inflammatory for joints and the digestive tract as well. Therefore, it is also good for fibromyalgia and IBS symptoms. It is healing to the tissues of the intestines, just as it is to the urinary tract.

Comfrey Root or Leaf - It's difficult to find the root, but usually you can find the leaf. Used to treat ulcers, this is a very healing herb that is best taken in a tea. Comfrey is soothing to the digestive tract and to all mucous membranes. I drank comfrey leaf tea along with marshmallow root tea to help heal my bladder lining. First I drank them separate, but later I would often add them together in a tea. I also used comfrey leaf in my herbal baths.

Cat's Claw (Una de Gato) - Excellent for boosting the immune system, Cat's Claw is also good for the intestines. I took one capsule of cat's claw a day along with drinking marshmallow root and comfrey tea. This way I was boosting my immune system and soothing my insides at the same time.

Echinacea/Goldenseal Liquid - Echinacea is a natural antibiotic and immune system stimulator. It's good for cleansing the blood and the lymph glands. Echinacea is used to treat bacterial infections, viruses, and yeast infections. Goldenseal is another natural antibiotic that also works against fungus. It works in the bloodstream to eliminate infection. It also boosts the immune system to fight infection and enhances the effectiveness of other herbs. Echinacea/Goldenseal in capsules is pretty strong for IC patients, which is why I recommend either making it in a tea or buying the liquid form. It can be taken under tongue or with water and you can take a lower dosage this way. I used to take 3-5 drops twice a day when fighting infection or the flu. It only works if you take it 7-10 days on and 7-10 days off. It is very important to take breaks or it will stop working. This is not something you want to take every day.

Mullein - While it is excellent for loosening mucous and congestion from the lungs, mullein also helps to strengthen the lymphatic system. Mullein is soothing to any inflammation and it also acts to reduce spasms. I would often dissolve part of a capsule using a small strainer in a cup of hot water. Sometimes I would dissolve part of a capsule right into my marshmallow root tea.

Raspberry Leaf - Very supportive to the female organs, raspberry leaf helps ease menstrual cramps and regulate menstrual flow. I drank a cup or two before and during my menstrual cycle every month.

Catnip - An anti-spasmodic that helps ease menstrual cramps, catnip is very relaxing. It is another herb that I drank in a tea during "that time of the month". I also drank catnip tea when I was trying to relax and get some sleep.

Sage - Among its many uses, sage also helps loosen mucous buildup. Sage tea is good for mouth sores and easing a sore throat. A purifying herb, I smoked it when I was quitting smoking, and added it to tea and to herbal baths.

Cinnamon - Good for infection, as a blood purifier, and digestive aid, cinnamon also enhances the effectiveness of other herbs. Some herbs are as simple as this...I ate it on cinnamon toast.

Ginger - Helps fight colds, flu, and infection. Like cinnamon, ginger enhances the effectiveness of other herbs. Though it is often used as a digestive aid, it's very strong to take internally for IC patients. One or two sips of plain ginger tea was sometimes helpful when I had the flu, but mostly it was excellent in the bath for pulling toxins out of muscles and joints.

Licorice Root - While helping balance the production of hormones, licorice root is also said to expel mucous from the respiratory tract. To me it was quite strong, so I would only drink one or two sips of the tea.

Peppermint Leaf - Good for soothing the stomach and aiding digestion. If your stomach is bloated with gas, a little peppermint tea will make you burp so you can feel better.

How to make herbal tea - I make herbal tea right in my drip coffee maker. It's quick and easy. You can make it with a tea ball, but I found this to be a pain in the neck and often the tea would be too strong. Remember, you don't have to make your herbal tea strong for it to work. Even after making the tea in the coffee maker, I would very often add ice cubes to cool it down and weaken it further. To make Marshmallow Root tea for example, I would use one heaping tablespoon of the root, to about 5 cups of water. The tea should not taste like much of anything. If it tastes bad, it's too strong. You can refrigerate the marshmallow tea if you want to. But keep in mind that just as regular iced tea gets stronger as it sits, so does herbal tea. Personally, this is why I didn't refrigerate it. Also, because it's so inexpensive and so easy to make, I would just make a new pot of tea the next time I was planning to drink it.

How to take an herbal bath - When my kidneys were inflamed and/or infected, I stayed away from taking really hot baths because it made my kidneys hurt worse. Therefore, most of the time that I was taking herbal baths, I was making them warm, rather than hot. In terms of temperature, do what you're comfortable with. The main reasons I used herbal baths was to pull toxins out of my body through my skin and/or to soothe and relax. (The skin being the largest eliminative organ in the body, I found this to be a mellow way to cleanse toxins out of my body without ingesting anything.) I put different "ingredients" in depending on what I was after.

I always started with a base of baking soda. I would start the water, then pour in about ¼ to a ½ cup of baking soda (by the way, I never measured). Then I would take a pinch or two of comfrey leaf (which is soothing and healing), sometimes parsley (which helps release water retention), and sometimes sage (which is a purifier). Most often I would use straight comfrey. Anyway, I would take whatever herbs I planned to use and put them in a tea ball that I would then throw into the tub. (This way you don't have little herbs floating around in the water with you. Yuck!) I usually used a small packet of herbal bath oil with vitamin E, which was soothing to the skin (and it smelled good too!). Then I would add one drop (sometimes two) of tea tree oil, which kills bacteria, fungus, and viruses, and this would be what would help pull toxins out of my skin. (The comfrey would be there to soothe the skin as the toxins were being pulled out by the tea tree oil. The baking soda would help neutralize the acids/toxins coming out.) If I was very congested I would put a drop of eucalyptus oil in the bath as well. At different times I added a drop of lavender or rose oil for fragrance (you can use any floral oil that feels right to you...I just liked the lavender and rose.) Sometimes I would add a couple drops of liquid echinacea/goldenseal to fight infection.

After throwing all this stuff in the bath, I would place two crystals in the tub with me. One was a black obsidian and the other was a rose quartz (though there were also times I used purple quartz). You do not have to use crystals in your herbal baths for the baths to work. I used them after learning about them because I felt they helped in my healing (and because I thought they were kind of cool). I chose the black obsidian to absorb all the negative stuff coming out of me in the bath. And the rose quartz to send love and healing energy through the water. I often burned either sage (which is purifying) or frankincense and myrrh incense (very healing scent) in the bathroom. I lit several candles and placed them around the tub and all around the bathroom. Then I turned off the lights and turned on some soothing mediation music and got in. I also had one of those soft blow up pillows for my head and body that went into the tub so that it would be more comfortable.

During my herbal baths, I tried to meditate and relax. I would picture the toxins and poisons leaving my body and being absorbed by the black crystal. I would picture the bathroom filling up with pink light coming from the rose quartz. I usually stayed in the tub around fifteen to twenty minutes, sometimes less, sometimes more. If I started to feel really crummy or something, I would get out. Brilliant huh? I did it by feel. There were several months where I took one to two herbal baths a day. I used to drink water while I was in the tub and when I got out.

Ginger baths are great for muscle and joint pain. When my fibromyalgia symptoms were severe, I often took a bath with one to two tablespoons of ginger. The ground ginger that you buy at the grocery store is perfect. Just stir it into a warm/hot bath. When I took a ginger bath, I put nothing else in the tub with it, just ginger. The ginger will pull toxins out of the muscles and joints. You will probably feel some pain when you first get in as the ginger is working, but when you get out, after being in the tub about ten minutes or so, you will feel much better. Again, drink a lot of water when you get out of the tub.

Essential oils are great for herbal baths. As I was saying earlier, I used a drop of eucalyptus oil in my herbal baths when I was congested. Sometimes I would just sniff it right from the bottle to clear my sinuses. And I often used one to two drops of tea tree oil in the bath to kill bacteria/fungus and help pull the toxins out through my skin. Tea tree oil is *very* strong and you barely need any of it for it to work. One drop is often plenty. I also used a tiny bit (less than a drop) of tea tree oil with water as a mouthwash/rinse to kill bacteria and help heal my gums. Some people rub a little lavender oil on their belly to help relieve pelvic/bladder pain. Also, a drop of peppermint oil on the temples is said to relieve headaches.

Meditation initially was very difficult. I had difficulty concentrating and relaxing when I was in so much pain and the constant urgency was certainly no help. But I bought a couple meditation tapes and just started turning them on. Even though I would have to get up after three minutes to go to the bathroom, I would just get back on the bed and rewind the tape. Sometimes I could only make it through a total of fifteen minutes trying to meditate. But eventually I was able to do a half hour without having to get up. It definitely got easier as I got better. And I got better at meditating too. It is not difficult to do. There are several healing meditation tapes on the market. Personally, I like Dick Sutphen's meditation tapes. I think he has a cool voice for getting you relaxed. Just turn on whatever tape you choose, listen, and do what they say. Often it is just the commitment of actually doing it every day that I think people find difficult. But it is definitely worth the effort in my opinion. Sometimes when you try to meditate, you may fall asleep. That's okay. It just means that your body needed the sleep. Whether you fall asleep or not, either way you are helping yourself get better. Meditation is a deep form of relaxation and is very healing to the body. If you don't choose to meditate or you find it too difficult, you might want to try the following before you go to sleep at night. Close your eyes and picture yourself healthy. Remember what it felt like to be healthy and strong. Visualize your healing. The power of the mind can be an amazing thing.

Relaxation is great for the immune system. Even if you just take a nap in the daytime, it will help so much. Rest is so important in healing. I know so many IC patients who don't treat themselves like they were sick. It's as if their bladder is sick, but the rest of them is not. So they continue to work, take care of the family, or run around doing whatever, thinking that it's good for them to stay active and involved. Maybe this is because everyone tells them they are not "sick" and that they will have this "defective" bladder the rest of their life, so they better learn to live with it. I do understand this way of thinking, especially for those who have mild to moderate IC. They assume they will have IC the rest of their lives and they aren't going to let it get the best of them. But in general, I disagree with this approach. Often all the stress from working and the constant activity is making the individual worse. And people with more severe IC symptoms are often so tense

147

from pain and fear that they find it difficult to relax, whether they have the "time" to or not. Very often IC patients are also getting very little sleep at night as well. Doing your best to relax and get as much rest as possible is very important in helping your body heal.

Some form of exercise is also important. Even a small amount that can get the lymph system moving will help. The lymph system does not have a pump the way the circulatory system has the heart to pump the blood through our veins and arteries. We have to help the lymph system flush itself and get the lymph fluids moving. This is one reason why some form of exercise is so important. It aids the body in its own healing processes. Whether you try yoga or walking, the rebounder or swimming, any form of exercise will do. At some point later in your healing you might be able to tolerate a lymphatic cleanser and rebuilder, but I would be careful with them initially. In the meantime, you can use more gentle approaches to cleanse and rebuild the lymph system without ingesting anything, such as using the rebounder or skin brushing, for example.

There is so much to be said about the mind/body/spirit connection when it comes to healing your body from IC, that I decided it should be the subject of another book. In the meantime, I definitely recommend reading about the mind/body/spirit connection. There are dozens of excellent books on the subject.

The following are some non-herbal products that I took. They are all non-toxic and gentle to the body, which, in my opinion, makes them very good options for IC patients.

Colostrum - Colostrum is found in mother's milk. Humans and cows both have Colostrum in their milk. The Colostrum I am referring to is taken from cows' milk immediately after the birth of a calf. These are organic, pasture-fed cows who are not given antibiotics or chemicals. Colostrum is full of immunoglobulins and therefore helps boost the immune system. It is a natural food product that kills bacteria, fungus, and viruses. And in this way it is also a cleanser. This is what I took while getting my fillings replaced to cleanse the mercury out of my body. I think I would have tried it earlier on if I had known about it. At the same time, I'm not sure if I would have been able to tolerate the cleansing it causes when I was really sick. However, I do believe it's an excellent choice for IC patients, in general, for several reasons. First because it's a natural antibiotic that doesn't kill off friendly bacteria and it works against fungus, viruses, and parasites, which, as far as I'm concerned, can all be involved in IC. Secondly, IC patients can't usually tolerate products that are harsh on the body. Where many cleanses are very harsh on the body, Colostrum is not. And lastly, Colostrum rebuilds as it cleanses. It boosts the immune system and aids the body in healing.

MSM - MSM stands for methyl sulfonyl methane. MSM is a non-metallic element found in every cell of every plant and every animal. Not to be confused with sulfa drugs, MSM is a "useable organic sulfur" and is a component of all living cells. It's a mineral that the body needs for healthy flexible cells. MSM is taken to help lots of different things. They say it helps with pain and inflammation and is good to help damaged cartilage in the joints, ligaments and tendons. It is also great for skin, hair and nails. It's supposed to help with allergies by helping the body flush out toxins and foreign substances more easily. MSM is said to coat mucousal surfaces and occupies the binding sites that could otherwise be used by challenging food allergens. It is also good for constipation. MSM is non-toxic and should be taken with Vitamin C. For IC patients, who usually can't tolerate vitamin C, they can take it with Ester C.

Flax Seed Oil - Great for the intestines and soothing to all mucous membranes, flax seed oil is also mellow to the body. You can use it where you might put butter or other oil on foods. I used to dribble it over brown rice. You can also buy it in capsule form. I used flax seed oil to help with my IBS symptoms.

Glucosamine Sulfate - Glucosamine Sulfate is fairly expensive. I bought mine in the bulk powder form because it was cheaper that way. I took this when my knees and other joints were most painful. I added the powder to my nutrition drink. When it felt as if the bones in my joints were rubbing against each other, this provided some type of "moisture" or lubrication and helped my knees and ankles a lot. There are several recent combination "drugs" that include Glucosamine Sulfate. Myself, I found that taking it alone was best. You may feel otherwise. As always, do what you think.

Aloe Vera Juice - I used to add it to a little kool-aid (and once I could tolerate it, I added it to juice). They make it in all kinds of flavors now. They also make freeze-dried aloe vera capsules, which personally I never tried, so I can't tell you if they will work as well as the juice. But I do know of many people who take the capsules, so if you can't stand the taste of the juice, you may want to try the capsules.

Ester C - As previously mentioned, most IC patients cannot tolerate citric acid or vitamin C. Also fairly expensive, Ester C is a non-acidic form of vitamin C that many IC patients find they can tolerate better.

Baking Soda - A major staple for the IC patient, in my opinion. I used it for so many things. Some IC patients drink a glass of water with a teaspoon of baking soda to ease burning during urination and pain in the bladder. (I could only tolerate drinking a few sips myself. But those few sips would help.) If you are using baking soda this way, be careful that 1) you don't have a sodium problem, and 2) that you don't overdo it because it can cause constipation if you take it too often. Baking soda helps flush the garbage out of you, while neutralizing the acid along the way. The ability of baking soda to neutralize acid makes it ideal for the IC patient. I put baking soda in my herbal baths as a base. I rinsed my mouth with baking soda and water to neutralize the mercury. After cleaning the tub or toilet with bathroom cleaner, I would use baking soda to re-wash them so that the chemicals would be neutralized and then they wouldn't bother me. When I had the rash on the back of my thighs from the bathroom cleaner, I put baking soda right on my skin to help absorb and neutralize the poisons/toxins coming out in the rash. When I got out of an herbal bath, I often put some baking soda in my hand and rubbed it lightly on my arms and legs, etc. to help absorb and neutralize the poisons/toxins coming out of my skin. When we moved into a new apartment and I was still very chemically sensitive, Charlie sprinkled baking soda all over and then vacuumed several times to neutralize the toxins coming from the new carpeting. We also set bowls of baking soda around the apartment to absorb all the odors coming from the new carpet. And on top of all of this, you can even use baking soda to make chocolate chip cookies!

These are all things to help balance the body. They are all non-invasive and you can do them yourself. Remember that treatments don't have to hurt to help.

I speak to so many IC patients who send me their regimen (what they do every day, what they take, etc.) and very often they are totally overdoing it. They are taking so many things that they can't possibly know which way is up; what is helping and what is hurting. With the element of allergies and the various symptoms that they cause (which differs individually), it is most likely that some of the things you are taking (especially in the form of synthetic medications) are in reality making you worse; throwing your body even more off balance. Some things you are taking may be putting even more of a strain on your immune system.

Sometimes it can get confusing when trying an herb or product that causes some form of cleansing to the body. Even if it is normally considered fairly mild cleansing, certain IC patients might still have a reaction. Even mellow things such as acidophilus, aloe vera juice, and Marshmallow Root, things that help many IC patients and things that I would normally recommend, even these, can cause a reaction in some people. For example, I know some IC patients who cannot tolerate acidophilus because they experience an increase in their Vulvodynia symptoms when they take it. And others who experience an increase

151

in their IBS symptoms when they take aloe vera or Marshmallow Root. Maybe they are allergic to it or maybe the cleansing or "flush" they cause is increasing their symptoms. It might also be that they are simply taking too strong a dose. The trick is knowing when you are cleansing and when you are hurting yourself. This is where getting to know your body is so important. And this is also why it is so important to go very slow when you first try something new.

It is my opinion that many IC patients who explore alternative treatments often overdo. They simply do too many things at the same time. IC patients are very sensitive and really have to go very, very slowly. Very often when people overdo it they are making themselves even more sick by rushing the poisons/toxins out of their body. They are being too hard on their bodies. You really have to give your body a chance to heal and not overwhelm it with too many things at once. This is so important and I really can't stress it enough. As you get to know your body, you will be better able to tell whether you are cleansing and it is a good thing or whether you are having a reaction to what you are taking and it is a bad thing. See if you can determine whether what you are doing for your IC right now is helping your body heal or making it more difficult for your body to heal.

*Remember to breathe...*

# Chapter 17

———◆———

# Physical Coping Tips

"Although the world is full of suffering, it is also
full of the overcoming of it."
- Helen Keller

Healing takes time and learning to cope during the healing process is very important. There are many, many things you can do to help yourself while you are healing from IC.

When I first started talking with my friend Cynthia about IC, one of the first things she told me was that I wasn't breathing. I was like WHAT? Of course I'm breathing. She said no. "You wait a long time in between breathing and when you do, you are taking small shallow breaths," she said. Then I realized that she was right. I rarely took a deep breath. Being in pain all the time, you might not realize that you aren't breathing "normally". You stop taking deep breaths because often they cause more pain. And then you get so use to it or pay so little attention to it that you don't even realize that you are no longer taking in much oxygen. Obviously oxygen is extremely important to the body and it's very important that we get enough of it to help us heal. Once I was aware, I had to make a concerted effort to remember to breathe. When the pain wasn't as severe, I would slowly practice taking deep breaths, holding them in, and then slowly letting them out. As often as I could think of it, I would stop what I was doing and take a deep breath. (Learning to meditate also helped me with learning to breathe again.) As silly and as simple as this advice may sound, I know it's as important to your healing as it was to mine. So…I tell you now what my friend told me. *Remember to breathe.*

Remember that old stupid joke where the patient says, "Doctor, doctor…it hurts if I go like this." And then the doctor says, "Then don't do that." For most IC patients, sitting or standing for long periods of time causes more pain and discomfort. So my advice…don't do that. For most IC patients, waiting too long to urinate causes more pain, sometimes nausea, and very often bladder spasms and "pee freeze". So my advice again…don't do that (as much as you can help it of course).

Keep logs to track your progress and to help you determine what is affecting you. For example, you might want to keep a frequency log (I kept mine in the bathroom with a clock next to it), a pain log, a medication log, and a food log. Keeping track of what you are taking, what you are eating, and how you are feeling is extremely helpful in determining whether your treatment approach is working for you. You also might want to keep your own medical records because you don't know how good of a job your doctor is doing. Get a copy of everything. For example, if you are having a cystoscopy, get a copy of the surgical report and a color copy of the inside of your bladder.

If you are new to all this and you are about to go in for a cystoscopy/hydrodistention, make sure you ask your doctor (and tell everyone you see before going into surgery) that you want the catheter removed BEFORE you wake up. This is the cause of so many people's nightmarish experience following cystoscopy. Some urologists mistakenly think this will help the patient. But instead, this can cause tremendous amounts of indescribable pain. So this is very important.

Decide if you like your doctor. Does he/she listen to you or answer your questions? If not, decide to get a new doctor. Better yet, decide to be your own doctor. Even if you are most comfortable having a urologist to treat your IC, you can still decide to be educated about IC and IC treatment options. You can still make your own informed decisions.

Pain medication should always be on hand. This is very important. Pain medication that you are not allergic to. Pain medication that you know works for you.

Make yourself as comfortable as possible. Whether it be mini-ice packs, heating pads, body pillows, extra pillows, extra soft toilet paper, whatever it takes. The pain, pressure, and urgency are uncomfortable enough. A good heating pad (or two) is especially important. Most IC patients have a heating pad permanently adhered to their bodies already, so this advice is not major news. Now they have heating pads that you can heat in the microwave and take with you in the car. Or you can get an ac adapter for the cigarette lighter in the car so you can plug one in there. Many IC patients who suffer from Vulvodynia symptoms recommend freezing a small can of tomato paste, in lieu of a mini ice pack, because it fits perfectly between the legs.

Make sure you keep lots of good reading material in the bathroom, because you will probably be spending an awful lot of time in there until you get better. I also found a portable phone to be an essential. It was the only way I could talk to anyone for any length of time. And there were so many emergency situations (like when I was passing kidney stones or having an allergic reaction to pain medication) where I was so incredibly grateful to have the phone there with me in the bathroom.

Avoid all acidic foods, alcohol, coffee, caffeine, chocolate, cranberry juice, lemon juice or any citrus fruit, tomatoes, spicy food, MSG, and any artificial sweetener. (I am always surprised to find IC patients who have no idea that they shouldn't be drinking wine or eating tomatoes. And it's very common for me to talk to IC patients who are still drinking soda or using artificial sweeteners.)

Keep a food diary to determine what foods cause you the most pain so that you can avoid them. We are all different when it comes to what foods we can tolerate, so it's important to determine which ones bother you. Don't just blindly follow a predetermined diet or you may end up hurting yourself without realizing it. It is important because of candida, and for many other reasons, to decrease not only the sugars in your diet, but the carbohydrates as well (since carbohydrates turn to sugar in the body). Very often IC patients have either a yeast or blood sugar imbalance, if not both.

After using an elimination diet or getting tested for allergies, you will be aware of what foods trigger your IC symptoms to get worse and then you can avoid them. An elimination diet is where you eliminate most everything and introduce foods one at a time, keeping a log to note symptoms, in order to determine which ones effect you negatively. A particular food can affect you right away after eating it, or anytime up to 24-48 hours afterward. So it's best to take a couple days in between before introducing something else.

Air purifiers or air cleaners are very helpful to keep germs, dust and other allergens out of the air. Avoid mold and mildew as much as possible. Especially if you find you have a problem with candida or are allergic to mold and mildew, because they may increase your symptoms.

Avoid chemical cleaners, paint fumes, strong perfumes (especially the cheaper ones that contain a lot of alcohol), and exhaust fumes, as much as possible. Especially avoid using chemical cleaners in your home. They make wonderful all natural cleaners now that are not harmful to the environment or you. I would also avoid using those toilet bowel cleaners that turn your water blue or green, such as with "drop-ins". I wouldn't use the clear ones with bleach either. As gross as it may sound, you don't want any to splash on you and you also want to be able to see the color of your urine. As many chemicals as you can avoid, whether they be in your environment or in your food, the better off you'll be.

Avoid scented and/or colored toilet paper. Avoid scented or deodorant menstrual pads. They make all natural cotton re-usable menstrual pads. I never tried them myself, but I know IC patients who swear by them, especially those with severe Vulvodynia symptoms. I would also avoid douches and tampons, especially the deodorant or extra absorbent kind.

Often the joke among IC patients is that we should buy stock in toilet paper companies. But I can assure you that I have no stock in Charmin when I tell you that Charmin with Aloe is the best. It is super gentle, but a bit more expensive than regular toilet paper. If you have irritation or Vulvodynia symptoms, I think it's great. You can also find Puffs with Aloe. (But first it is a good idea to find out if you are allergic to aloe or it will aggravate your Vulvodynia symptoms, rather than help them. You can always try it and see how you do.) Also for irritation, you can use a small squirt bottle with warm water and a soft cotton towel to pat dry.

Speaking to other IC patients is one of the smartest things we can do. Not only for the emotional support and understanding that we can provide each other, but for the exchange of knowledge and experiences. If you can't find a local support group meeting or physically can't make it to one, see if you can get on line and talk to IC patients through the computer. As I said earlier in the book, the computer was a major life savor for me because, at the time, there was no local support group in my area. And even if there were, physically, I would never have been able to attend. If you don't have a computer, maybe you can go to the library and use one there. The Internet is an excellent way to keep abreast of the current research on IC.

For when you can't start the urine stream…take deep breaths to relax and try not to push at first. I know the instinct is to push and that's what I always used to do. But then I learned that the reason nothing would come out was because of bladder spasms, so relaxing your bladder (and yourself) as much as you can will really help. Here is a technique Charlie invented for me. He would sit in the other room and say this to me as I sat waiting and trying not to panic. He would say, "Close your eyes and picture your feet relaxing. Now feel your calves relaxing. Now feel your thighs relaxing…and your bladder…on up through your body." (Can you tell Charlie has listened to my meditation tapes with me?) So I used that technique all the time. No matter where I was, I would close my eyes and start relaxing my body from the feet up. Another thing to help relax the bladder is to use a warm washcloth and hold it over your bladder and on your vagina. I know some people who use a small squirt bottle with warm water in it. You can try to have water running in the bathroom, though sometimes this is a form of torture. You can see if it works for you. There are also acupressure points that you can press right in the middle of your temples. They are "flush" points and this also helped me a lot with "pee freeze". But most importantly, try hard to relax and try not to panic.

For when it burns to urinate or you get sharp shooting pains you can use medications such as Pyridium or Urised. (Obviously, you have to be able to tolerate them. These medications help some IC patients and not others.) Drink lots of distilled water to dilute the urine. Taking Prelief or some kind of antacid like Rolaids, Tums, or Tagamet to reduce acid is also helpful for many IC patients. As an alternative, I would suggest drinking marshmallow root tea and/or aloe vera juice. Take pain medication and/or a muscle relaxant (anti-spasmodic) for the sharp, shooting pains. Use the heating pad immediately after voiding to help the spasms (I used to call these aftershocks).

Very often, the first time you urinate in the morning can be especially painful. This is usually because that's when your urine is the most toxic and your bladder the most full. I used to dread that first time in the morning! So what I did was take Pyridium at night shortly before going to bed, so that it would still be in my system by morning. I would be very careful what I ate and drank in the evenings, before bed. The more acidic the food or the more irritating the drink, the more it would hurt in the morning. Even if I took Pyridium, drank only water, and ate bland food, the first time urinating in the morning was usually still the most painful and difficult. But paying attention to these few things definitely helped.

For when you have to ride in the car you can put foam (like from a mattress pad) or a pillow under your feet on the floor, and/or on the seat and seat back, to help absorb the vibrations as much as possible. Try to locate all the bathrooms ahead of time, so you know when you can stop. This will cut down on the stress of not knowing when you can get to a bathroom. Have your I Can't Wait card from the ICA or a medic alert bracelet to show if you are someplace in public that doesn't have a public restroom. This way store employees, for example, will understand that you have a medical condition that causes you to HAVE to use the bathroom right away. Avoid long car rides as much as you can. Bring something to "go" in, in case of emergency in the car, which will also help reduce the stress of not knowing where the next bathroom is. I know some IC patients who use a big Ziplock baggie and others who use a plastic storage container with a lid. Try to avoid car rides with people who don't understand that you need to stop NOW, not in 5-10 minutes.

For when you have to go somewhere in public or to a friends...be honest about your IC. There is nothing to be ashamed of about saying that you have IC and have to use the bathroom frequently. I know some IC patients who try to hide their IC from friends, co-workers, and even family/relatives. Whether from embarrassment or from not feeling like explaining and then possibly having them not understand, this happens more often than I would have initially thought. Those who have more severe IC have most likely gotten past the point of having anything embarrass them anymore. I know one woman who said she could probably pee in the middle of a stadium full of people. I don't know if I could do that, but I'm certainly less shy than I ever was before.

161

# Chapter 18

◆

# Emotional Coping Tips

*"Every problem has a gift for you in its hands."*
*- Richard Bach*

My first day on line after getting diagnosed was very informative and affirming. It was such a relief to know that I wasn't alone. I was not the only person in the world that had been treated this way. Before this whole experience I could never have imagined being treated this way by doctors, friends, co-workers, etc.. I would have never guessed that anything like this could happen to me. It's very bizarre to get treated like you're "crazy" when you're not. It's very frustrating (to say the least), and personally, I found it pretty insulting. Just knowing how many perfectly sane, intelligent women out there have had this same experience helped me to not take it personally. Like any other person with a serious illness, there are many emotions IC patients are forced to deal with. Getting through these emotions is part of healing.

I believe there are four main psychological effects of having IC. Fear, I think, is number one. The fear of not getting better. The fear of wondering if you will ever be "you" again. Plus, IC can really be quite a scary disease. IC patients often have all kinds of mysterious symptoms, drug reactions, and other severe allergic reactions. Often the doctors don't know what is going on, in terms of the cause of the symptoms, which also makes it scary. Often we have to deal with these "reactions" and strange symptoms on our own. Anger is second. Anger at having IC. Anger at the people in our life who don't understand. Anger at the doctors who have treated us poorly. There is a lot of anger that IC patients experience. Thirdly there is guilt. We can't do the things we used to do and we have to say no to so many things and so many people. Many of us feel we are disappointing our loved ones. Shame is the last major one. Many people who have IC have been made to feel that they are somewhat responsible for having it. Many are embarrassed to let people know they even have IC. These four things are not easy to deal with. It is important to talk to someone about all these feelings. I know so many IC patients who are very depressed. It's understandable, of course, because having IC can be a miserable experience, often with seemingly no end in site. If you are depressed and/or considering suicide, please find yourself someone to talk to. There is no shame in asking for help dealing with the effects of having IC.

*My #1 coping tip...allow yourself to cry.* Having IC taught me to allow myself to be however I want, which wasn't an easy thing for me to learn. If I was upset or feeling sick of being so sick or in that I'm-in-a-lot-of-pain-and-about-to-loose-my-mind state, I would just let myself feel bad. Not forever, but for a little while. I think it's important to allow ourselves to feel bad sometimes. I mean, for the most part, I think I've had a pretty great attitude about all of this. The IC, the pain I've been through, the way I've gotten treated by other people because of IC, the not being able to have sex with my beautiful husband for seemingly endless periods of time, etc.. But when I don't have that great attitude, I no longer feel guilty about it. There's no reason to apologize or feel bad about feeling bad. We have every right to feel bad after what we go through with IC. We often talk a lot about having a good attitude when it comes to getting better, the importance of believing that we will get better, etc., but it is also important to remember that it's okay to feel bad sometimes. It's natural, normal, and well deserved. When you feel bad...let yourself cry, scream, and complain.

Crying is a release and is very healing. Screaming, whining, complaining, bitching, crying...these are all ways to get out the frustration and anger, the pain and the fear. It is much healthier to get it out of you then it is to keep it in. Talk to someone who really cares and who will listen to you with love. Then do something to completely make yourself happy. Anything. Whatever makes you the most happy. Cheer yourself up somehow. Spoil yourself, because you deserve it. This is definitely one way I coped.

Another way I chose to cope was to spend a few minutes every day writing down everything I was grateful for. Just because we're allowed to be crabby and upset, doesn't mean we can't, at the same time, be grateful for what we do have. There are always other people out there who have it worse. I have found that most IC patients just naturally appreciate every little thing; all the small things in life that other people normally take for granted. Because for many of us, there are a lot of things we couldn't do for a long time. We sure do learn to appreciate things when they are taken away. Even at my worst I was thankful to find other IC patients on line that I could talk to. I was thankful to have a computer to talk to them through and from the privacy and comfort of my own bedroom no less. I was one of the lucky ones. This disease was even more lonely and difficult to deal with before the advent of the Internet, and for some today, it still remains just as lonely.

Loneliness is something that many IC patients may have to deal with. Many times we feel "left out". Maybe we can't attend family functions or holidays because of the long car ride or because of how we're feeling. Maybe we can't go to the party or the baseball game or out to dinner, etc. It can be very difficult to plan anything with an IC patient. Every day can be different. Even within one day, things can change dramatically. Maybe you are doing okay in the morning and by evening you feel completely awful and absolutely can't go out as planned. This can be difficult for other people to understand.

Many IC patients find that they lose friends after getting sick. I remember how I had to tell one "friend" that I couldn't be in her wedding anymore because I was too sick and she never spoke to me again. Others said I would never get better and wanted nothing more to do with me. Still others thought I was crazy, exaggerating, or simply didn't want to take the time to understand. There will probably be people in your life who don't understand and normally well-meaning people who will say stupid things to you. This is just one of those things that comes with having IC.

I think that dealing with the people in our lives who don't understand IC is very difficult. I know that this was something that I had a problem with. It took me a while to understand, but eventually I realized that we basically have three choices here. We can choose to disregard these people. In a sense, cut them out of our life (for lack of a nicer way of saying it). We can take the time and energy to try to get them to understand what we're going through. Or lastly, we can just decide to accept them for who they are in the moment, recognizing that they may not be ready to understand. Maybe they are afraid to know what IC is. Some people are afraid of illness that they don't understand and they don't even like to think about it or talk about it. Or maybe the fact is that they just don't really care. It's very difficult when the people who don't understand are the people that we love and want in our lives. To me, those are the people to spend the time and energy trying to "explain" IC to. At the same time, my advice is to let go of those people who don't "want" to understand right now. Stand up for yourself with those you really care about. And know that it's okay. It is not your fault you have IC.

I think that we also need to realize the way the rest of the world seems to view IC. I have spoken to a lot of people (non-IC patients) about this and I asked them what they think other people think IC is all about. I learned that the general public doesn't seem to think IC is that big a deal. They haven't heard of it on television or the radio. There aren't any books about it. Nobody they know has died from it. The medical profession hasn't exactly given it tons of attention. So basically there is a general lack of interest where the majority of people are concerned. When it comes to the people we are close to (family and friends), those people are the toughest to deal with when they don't show understanding. It is hurtful and can make us feel like they don't care about us, even when that might not really be the case.

You know how they say that when you're rich and successful that it's difficult to know who your friends are? Well, when you have IC, you know *for certain* who your friends are. In general, we need to allow ourselves to not care what other people think of us. People need to accept us for who we are, with IC or without. And often with IC, you can't fake it. You might have to accept that you can't eat what they are serving for the holiday dinner, or maybe that you can't go on that long car ride to join them for the evening, or maybe you can't walk up and hug them hello because it will hurt. You just can't worry about what "they" will think. I'll tell you what Charlie always used to tell me...*relax into yourself.* Just let yourself be. And know that it's okay.

*The irony of the name IC is that no one can see it.* No one can see the pain or the inside of your bladder. Many IC patients look "normal" and often do not appear "sick" (especially those with mild to moderate IC). IC patients get use to being in pain and doing things in pain. So often people don't even realize that we are in pain because we act and look "normal". When my IC was severe, I looked deathly ill and didn't have to deal with this problem. But as I was getting better, I did. I started to look more "normal" and even when I was in pain, no one could tell unless I complained. And I didn't complain much. At least initially I didn't complain much. Not until I learned that crying and complaining was all part of my healing.

IC can be a devastating illness that affects every part of your life. Often doctors don't even validate the IC patient's pain and symptoms, which further causes spouses and/or family to minimize what the patient is going through. If a spouse and/or family member hears a doctor minimizing IC as an illness, it can have a HUGE negative effect on the

167

IC patient's life. I have heard horror stories from IC patients about their spouses showing no understanding at all of what they were going through, blaming them for being sick or for having to go to the bathroom so often. I have heard of spouses who won't even give the IC patient privacy in the bathroom so that they can relax and get their bladder to work or they won't pull over when they're in the car so the person can go to the bathroom. This can cause a lot of discomfort and pain for the IC patient, to not be able to go when they need to. It breaks my heart to hear these things from people. I always try to get them to show their spouse articles on IC or *something* to get them to understand.

Also, I have heard from so many IC patients who have sex simply to please their partners. No matter how much pain or discomfort it causes them, they do it anyway. And this is not just pain during, it's painful for hours and days afterward. When I hear this from people, it makes me feel so sad. We need to be honest with our spouses. Remember that when it hurts, you don't have to have sex! There are other ways to satisfy your spouse without hurting yourself in the process. Sex should be pleasurable. It is an expression of love. If you are not aware of other ways to "please" your spouse, there are definitely ways to learn. It can even be fun! Even if you can't have sex, there are ways you can make each other feel good. At the same time, it is important to remember that our spouses need to feel desired. And because we love them, and let's face it, because we miss it, sometimes we go for it anyway. In those instances, we can do things like use K-Y Jelly or other lubricants. Try various positions to try to (excuse the expression but) find a comfortable fit without really hurting our bladders too much. The most important thing I want to stress is that there are other ways to sexually satisfy your spouse and you can even make them fun. But when you are in pain and feeling really lousy…hey…he's just going to have to understand. If he loves you…he will.

I wanted to be able to offer some advice to people who love an IC patient. I thought to myself, what could I say to help them deal with the frustration and helplessness of watching someone they love suffer so much. I decided to ask Charlie what he would tell someone who was in his position. Here is his advice. First and foremost, remember that it could just as easily be you. And if it was you, wouldn't your spouse be taking care of you right now? Remember to have patience because the IC patient can't help that they have IC. Remember that people in pain (who get very little sleep) don't always think clearly. They may say things that they don't mean. Remember that you can't solve the problem (IC), but you *can* listen to them and let them complain. You can be there for them by showing concern and love, taking them to their doctor appointments, being supportive of their treatment choices, and helping to explain to other people who don't understand. You will be helping just by being there, just by loving them the same way you did before they got sick. And last but not least, you can help them to eliminate stress in their lives so that they can have a better chance of getting better.

Not only does IC teach you who your friends are and who really cares about you, it also teaches you to care about yourself. In order to get better, you need to care about yourself. Maybe you are like me and need to learn to be nicer to yourself and put yourself first for a change. Or maybe you need to slow down and your IC is forcing you to do that.

Having IC can certainly cause you to look at yourself differently and/or feel that others do. Maybe we think of ourselves as "broken" or "damaged". We can't have sex, can't work, can't go places, can't do the things we used to do. We are not able to do or be what we once were. We have been told a lot of stupid things by doctors and maybe some of them have made us doubt ourselves or our sanity. Depending, of course, on how severe your IC (and IC-related symptoms) are, you might at times feel useless (can't work, can't take care of the house/family), feel like a burden to one who loves you, feel like a bubble-child (home all the time), feel like you're disappointing others, feel lonely, scared, angry, frustrated. Sometimes, remembering who we were before IC, what we were once able to do without a second thought, can make us sad/upset/angry. Okay, now that I have you all depressed!

I happen to believe that in every experience in life, there is a lesson (sometimes many) and a chance for growth of the "self" or soul. IC is certainly one of those experiences. IC forces us to make changes or adjustments in our lives. I believe this is one of the positives about IC. I have learned a lot about myself on my path of healing from IC. And I believe that it is ALL part of healing. The adjustments or changes I have made in my life and the lessons I had to learn, may not be the same as yours, but maybe mentioning some of mine can help you to recognize your own. One of the most major things I've learned is to be nicer to myself. Something that helped me a lot was when Charlie got upset one day as I was talking down about myself and he grabbed a pen and paper and wrote "I count" really big on the paper. Then he hung it up on the wall in the bedroom right above the computer where I would see it all the time. The sign stayed up on the wall for several months, until it finally sunk in. I had always taken care of everyone else before me. I don't do that anymore. I learned to eliminate stress from my life (as much as possible, of course) because stress isn't good for my immune system or my happiness. I've learned to stand up for myself in many different ways. I know how I feel physically and no one can tell me different. I've learned to listen to my body, to be sensitive to what it needs/wants…and then to act on it, as opposed to ignoring it. I was always so healthy and active; I never HAD to pay attention before. I've learned to have more faith in myself and to trust myself more. IC made me look at myself, which helped me to grow and to heal.

# Finding Your Path...

# Chapter 19

---◆---

# Now what do you do?

Okay…so now what do you do?

The first thing to address is the pain. Not every IC patient has pain as a symptom, but if you are in pain, do anything you can to get out of it. Pain is draining to your immune system and will almost feed on itself. The pain of IC can be excruciating and relentless. It keeps you from sleep that you desperately need. If you have nothing to take for pain, try to find a pain doctor or pain clinic. Because, as I've mentioned, very often urologists refuse to prescribe pain medication for their IC patients, it is often necessary to find a doctor who specializes in treating pain. Though I am not recommending it, I do know people who have called friends or relatives to get their old pain medications. And though I never did this, I certainly can relate to that type of desperation. I also know several IC patients who smoke marijuana as a muscle relaxant (great for bladder spasms) and as a pain reliever. Marijuana also helps with nausea and sleep. What I'm saying here is *do whatever you have to do*. You don't deserve to be in pain. No one does. This is often where I hear other IC patients say things like they wish they had cancer instead of IC. At least then someone would care. At least then they could get something for the pain. It is really quite tragic and I know so many people who have felt that way. In fact, the pain of IC has been likened to cancer pain. The only difference is that most doctors don't recognize it as such.

The next thing to address is the most prevailing symptoms, which often are the bladder symptoms. Do whatever you can to soothe your bladder. Adjust your diet. Determine what foods irritate you the most. Don't just blindly follow a predetermined diet, because remember, we are all different when it comes to what foods we can tolerate. Whether you take Pyridium, Urised, or drink aloe vera juice and/or Marshmallow Root tea, it's important to do things to soothe your bladder. Do anything you can to help your bladder to deal with all the garbage coming out through the urine. Drink lots of distilled water to dilute your urine and reduce the acid and toxicity.

Come up with a plan of attack (so to speak) on your IC. First I would try to figure out how you got IC. Try to think back to when your symptoms first began. Try to remember what changed at that time. Did you do anything different, were you exposed to anything new, did you drink or eat anything different, did you have surgery, dental work, a bladder infection, etc.. This might help you to figure out what may be involved in your particular situation. Even if you've had IC for years, this can still be helpful. Maybe when you think back, you will remember things or think of things that you never thought of before.

The following are some other things you might want to consider when deciding on what you think IC is and what treatment method is appropriate for you. For example, in terms of allergies and their role in your IC and IC related symptoms, I would consider the following. If your IC began immediately following your first sexual experience and if you used condoms or an IUD, consider that you might have a latex allergy and that it may have been a contributing factor in your IC. If your IC began immediately following surgery with a catheter, consider that you may have an allergy to latex. If your IC began immediately following dental surgery or dental work, consider that you may have an allergy to mercury and/or latex. If you have jaw pain or TMJ, earaches and sinus problems, problems with your teeth and gums, burning tongue, receding gums, or blisters in your mouth, consider that you might be allergic to mercury. If you have crowns in your mouth or have had a root canal, consider that mercury may play a role in your IC. You

174

might also want to consider whether an allergic reaction may have spurred your susceptibility to the IC bacteria....or to IC (however you want to look at it). *You might want to consider being tested for allergies before succumbing to treatments that involve latex being inserted into your body.*

I would also try to decide whether you believe that IC is an infection or not. Did your IC begin with repeated bladder infections or one huge bladder infection? Did your IC begin immediately following surgery? Did you have an infection immediately following your surgery? Do your other symptoms appear like an infection (fever, swollen glands, etc.)? You might want to consider having your urine cultured using a more sophisticated broth culturing technique. If you do believe IC is an infection, then you can decide if you want to fight it with antibiotics and anti-fungal medication or if you want to take herbs and use "alternative" methods to help your body to fight it. Many people seem to concentrate on killing the bacteria (or the fungus and parasites which often accompany IC) and forget how important it is to build up the immune system so that our bodies can kill the bacteria by themselves. Taking synthetic antibiotics often further perpetuates the problem. Maybe you kill one organism and others will replace it. Or maybe it will mutate further and become more antibiotic resistant. At the same time you might also want to consider that antibiotics will be throwing your body even more off balance than it already is by creating a perfect environment for yeast to thrive and by further weakening your immune system. What I'm trying to say here is that if you decide to take synthetic antibiotics, remember to replace the good bacteria that is being killed by taking a lot of acidophilus. (Don't forget to wait a few hours between taking the antibiotic and taking the acidophilus or you will be inhibiting the effects of the antibiotics.) Try to keep your body in balance. I would also do things to boost your immune system, because the antibiotics are tough on your immune system as well.

You might want to think about the role that candida may already play in your IC symptoms. Have you taken repeated antibiotics? Have you taken birth control pills or steroids? Do you crave sugar and breads? When you look in the mirror at your tongue is it coated with a white film? Do you get repeated vaginal yeast infections? You might want to consider taking a candida quiz or being tested for systemic yeast. (You will probably have to go to an alternative type of healer for this as most medical doctors do not regard candida as a real issue.)

If you decide that IC is a bladder disease (not systemic) and desire to treat the bladder with instillations, be aware of the side effects and risks involved. Ask other IC patients about bladder instillations before trying them. And remember to ask for pediatric size catheters and pain medication (or at least urethra numbing medications) before the instillation.

If you decide to treat your whole body, know that at different stages, different treatments are appropriate. Try to determine where you are in the moment with your IC. It is the first step in figuring out how to bring balance back into your body and into your life.

*Bringing your body back into balance is the way to heal from IC.* Giving your bladder and your body what it needs to give it a chance to heal. The actions can be the same no matter what perspective about IC you might be coming from. Whether you view IC as bacteria, bacteria and fungus, acid, toxins, poisons, or all of these, it doesn't matter so much. Whether you view IC as an autoimmune disease or a connective tissue disease, an allergic reaction or something hormonal, it doesn't matter much either. As long as you recognize that your whole body is involved and you "treat" your whole body, you can get well. The actions can be basically the same. In any of those cases, you can recognize that your body is out of balance. Hormones are out of balance, the healthy intestinal flora is out of balance (i.e., candida), the blood sugar may be out of balance; the immune system is suppressed and/or over-worked. All of these are typically the case with IC. Obviously our bodies are not functioning "normally". Our bodies have become sensitive to everything around it and everything we put into it. So be careful of both.

*Be nice to your body.* Give yourself rest, relaxation and no stress. Don't let people talk you into taking a whole bunch of garbage. The more stuff you take, the harder it is on your body. *Soothe your insides, gently cleanse out the toxins, rebuild and boost your immune system, in whatever ways you are most comfortable with.*

There are many, many ways to release toxins from the body using "alternative" methods. Gentle alternatives. That's the key. Be gentle with yourself. The more toxic you are, the more gentle you need to be while cleansing the toxins out. Once your body is out of balance it is not always so easy to get it back into balance. Sometimes doing a cleanse, you can cause other imbalances if you do it too much. So be careful that you are not over-cleansing. You want to gently rebuild while you're cleansing and more forcefully rebuild following a cleanse. If you cleanse too much, you will strip the body of needed nutrients, electrolytes, and minerals.

For example, you are not going to want to do something like NAET and an anti-candida program at the same time. Both are cleansing to the body. That would be overdoing it. You would be better to cleanse with one thing and soothe with others, boosting your immune system the whole way along. And if you're going to have your mercury fillings replaced, for example, you really have to go slowly, one tooth at a time, because you will have a lot of poisons to process in between. The more you do at once, the harder it is on your bladder and the rest of your body. The same with NAET treatments, at the most, you want to be treated for only one allergen a week. Take the time in between to allow your body to adjust to the treatment and flush out the toxins.

Remember that it takes time and that you will not necessarily see results as quickly as you would like. (Which would be like today...right?) If you are in a situation right now where you can't tolerate taking much of anything, you can start out with just drinking a lot of water to gently flush the body. Or you can try herbal baths if you can tolerate the water pressure. Something else you can try is to just sit on a rebounder without bouncing, just for a minute or two. There are many things you can try where you don't ingest anything, yet you will still be helping yourself.

*Your body is already trying to heal itself.* I believe that just as we, as humans, have an instinct to survive, our bodies have an "instinct" to heal. I believe our bodies are already trying to heal themselves. Whether the body or immune system is reacting to bacteria, candida, a specific allergen or various allergens simultaneously, or even to poisonous mercury, I believe it is most definitely reacting to something. Let's look at IC. Let's listen to our bodies. I believe our symptoms are talking to us. Our bodies always talk to us and tell us what they need. Take pain, for example, pain is not an illness; it's a symptom of illness. Pain is there to tell us that something is wrong. It is our body "speaking" to us. Rather than viewing IC symptoms as some mysterious attack on the body, I see them more as a form of protection. Our bodies are trying to rid themselves of bacteria/fungus/toxins/acids. This is where the frequency, urgency, and irritation are coming from. It's the bladder saying, "Get this stuff OUT OF HERE!"

Trying to prevent and/or stop the natural protection mechanisms of the body is not always such a good idea. Bladder holding protocol is a good example. If there is a toxic substance or an unseen, unidentified bacteria in the urine, holding the urine in the bladder for great lengths of time may not be such a great idea. If the body is telling us to get it out, I say, get it out. Another example is taking anti-histamines to stop the body from producing more mast cells (or histamines). This may not be such a great idea either if we look at it from the perspective that our bodies are producing those mast cells for a reason. Mast Cells are present in mucous tissues in the body, where you are likely to come into contact with foreign material or toxic chemicals, the nose or sinuses, the mouth, the bladder, the intestines. It is no wonder that IC bladders frequently have abnormal numbers of mast cells. Between allergic reactions, toxic mercury, bacteria, and fungus, how could there

178

not be. The mast cells are there for protection. That's their job. And to inhibit them, though it may mask symptoms temporarily, may cause more harm in the long run or may make it more difficult for your body to heal.

Try to always have another treatment idea on the sidelines in case what you're doing isn't working. There will be setbacks. Believe me....I had HUGE setbacks along the way. But healing IS possible, no matter how bad your bladder is right now. And that's why I write this book. So that you know it's possible. So that you know that the medical way is not the only way to treat IC. So that you know there are alternatives.

# Chapter 20

———◆———

# Taking Your Power Back

In my opinion, there are only certain things that medical doctors know how to do for us. They give us pills to cover symptoms, they run tests, do surgery, and then give us more medication. I strongly believe that they are often, unintentionally of course, causing more harm to the IC patient.

IC patients are overly toxic and often doctors are giving them medication after medication. Is this not adding to their toxicity? Maybe one medication is working to cover symptoms, but then the effects wear off (which is what usually happens). Then the IC patient switches medications or takes another one for another symptom and on and on. Often these medications are making the situation worse. Sometimes even the patient recognizes this, but continues to take the medication! They stay on it because the doctor tells them to and/or because they don't know what else to do. They are told that it takes a long time for the medication to work, so they have to stay on it a long time to see if it will help them or not (which I'm sure is the case with certain medications). And so they are a "bad patient" if they stop taking it. They are looked at funny by friends and family because if they are in SO much pain, why are they not doing what the doctor tells them to do. So they go against their better judgment and continue on taking the pills that are not only not working, but may even be making them worse. This happens a lot. Whether it be with bladder coating drugs, antibiotics, tricyclic anti-depressants, anti-histamines, or anti-spasmodics...I've seen it happen with them all.

I know many IC patients who feel very victimized by urologists and doctors in general. They feel very vulnerable. They will say things like "we are at the mercy of the doctor" and "what else are we to do?". They feel they don't have a choice in the matter. Even if they are very uncomfortable about a treatment or procedure, they will often go ahead with it anyway. They feel they must do what their doctor says even if they know that it's hurting them or making them worse.

*Learn to listen to your self.*
It's funny...sometimes I actually consider myself lucky for having all the horrendous experiences I had with doctors prior to getting diagnosed. Mostly because it's one of the things that pushed me, right away, into taking control of my own treatment. I think otherwise I would have trusted the doctors more, instead of myself. As previously mentioned, I know there are some of you who have doctors that you like, who listen to you, and who are open to options, etc., which is wonderful. But I also know that there are many of you out there who aren't so lucky. A major frustration of having IC is finding a doctor who cares and who will take the time. But in either case, whether you like your doctor or not, it is still very important to research your own treatments. Do not just trust the doctor to know what is best for you. Remember that you know your body better than any doctor could. Just because your doctor wants you to try a certain medication or bladder instillation, doesn't mean that it's the smartest thing for you to do. There may be side effects that your doctor is unaware of...even long term side effects to consider that he may not have mentioned. Even if you like your doctor and think he/she is terrific, he may be honestly unaware of the treatment repercussions, whereas other IC patients can usually tell you how it really is. Ask other IC patients about their experiences with a particular treatment before you try it. Even though we are all different, you will still gain valuable insight into treatments and side effects from other IC patients.

*Have faith in yourself.*
Have faith in that feeling you get in your gut. The feeling you get when you "just know" that something is right for you....or wrong for you.

Having blind trust in any healer or physician is not wise. It is wise to trust yourself first. Getting advice is wonderful. Having a caring, compassionate, skilled physician is also wonderful. But knowing when something isn't right for you and then acting on your own advice is the best.

*Learn to listen to your body.*
So how do you learn to listen to your body? There are a couple things to point out here. First you can start to pay closer attention to your symptoms. How do you feel in the morning versus the afternoon or evening? What changed when you first started feeling a certain way? What did you eat? What changed in your environment? What changed for you with regard to stress or emotions? What are the changes you are feeling in your body? *Notice how you are feeling.* This is very important. I know that IC patients often do this naturally because we have so many aches and pains that we have no choice but to notice them. But what I mean is to keep a log. Write it down so that you'll remember so that you can notice the subtle changes. There is also listening to your body when it comes to what you are craving to eat, where you are having pain, where your skin is breaking out, etc.. Using acupressure points or reflexology can also help you to learn a lot about what is going on in your body.

*Make sure you feel comfortable with what you're doing to your body.*
I'll say it again...trust yourself. And know that there are other options and other doctors available to you if you decide you are uncomfortable with your doctor's treatment suggestion. Taking charge of your own treatment definitely takes effort. I know it's not easy to do all this research while you're feeling so awful and it would sure be a lot easier to just trust your doctor to make all these decisions for you and hope that he/she is doing all the necessary research, etc., but it's just probably not smart where IC treatment is concerned. Just remember to do only what feels right to you. Whether it's medications or herbs, whether it's acupuncture or bladder instillations, you have to be the one to decide and to feel comfortable with what you're doing to your body.

*Eliminate stress and get enough rest.*

It's all about getting your life and your body back in balance. However you can do that. It will be different for everyone. Write down everything in your life that stresses you out and try to eliminate as many as you possibly can. Stress, I assure you, will make you much worse. You can probably notice that every time you are under stress there is an immediate difference in your physical body. And when you have IC, the symptoms are very dramatic. When I was under stress, I would feel nerve type pain down the backs of my arms coming from my neck and the back of my head. I wouldn't be able to urinate at all. I would feel sick to my stomach and get serious poison rushes. My body temperature would also react. I would lose some of the feeling in my hands from the nerve pain coming down the back of my arms. All kinds of things would happen immediately upon getting upset or really stressed out. You may have to learn to draw the line with certain people. You may have to learn to say no. Even to yourself. Talk with your spouse/significant other and/or family and ask for their help in eliminating the stressful things on your list. There is nothing wrong with asking for help eliminating your stress. You can explain to your loved ones how the stress is affecting you physically. Stress will always exacerbate IC symptoms. And why not? Stress makes all illnesses worse. Stress lowers the immune system and makes everyone more susceptible to illness. If this is true for every other disease, you can be quite sure that it is true for IC. You have to be willing to make the necessary changes to get well. If you stay in a stressful state, it will make it much more difficult to get better.

It's hard to feel strong when you're sick and in pain. I understand that. I wasn't used to crying before I got sick. And then there I was, crying every time I woke up, crying during the night, crying in the bathroom, crying out of frustration, pain, and fear. I would tell Charlie that I couldn't believe how much I was crying all the time and that I didn't used to be like that. And there he would be telling me how brave I was. I would say "What?! I'm not brave. I cry all the time. I'm scared all the time. Even when I don't act like it, I'm still scared." "That's okay," he would tell me. "You are still dealing with this. You are still researching all the time and trying to get better. You are not giving up. And that takes courage. So you see...you are brave." But I didn't feel so brave. Mostly I felt afraid and angry. Angry that I got IC in the first place. Angry at the doctors and people who hurt me. Angry at myself, mostly, for letting them. So I took that anger I felt and put it to good use. I used it to take my power back. And now I realize that it's the first step. If you want to get better from IC, it's almost as if you have no choice. You need to take your power back so that you can begin to heal.

Why me?
There was something that my dad used to say to me when I was growing up that I'll always remember. He used to tell me that if you were going to ask God "Why me?" when bad things happened, then it was only fair to ask Him "Why me?" when good things happened. Maybe we don't understand the reason why things happen, but true faith is knowing that there are still reasons. That everything that happens is for our highest good, whether we understand it at the time, or not. So many people have asked me how I was able to keep such a great attitude while I was sick. There were several reasons, not the least of which was the love Charlie and I share. But another reason was something else my dad always taught me. "As a man thinketh in his heart, so is he." What you believe is what you draw to you. It is one of the laws of the universe. Thoughts are things, he would tell me. Thoughts are things. *Believe you will get well.*

You can do this. I know you can.

...remember to breathe

# References

[1] Health Force. Robert Lewanski and Robert E. Zuraw, Waterford, MI, 1982, p.10.

[2] Boyd, N.D., Benediktsson, H., Vimy, M.J., Hooper, D.E., and Lorscheider, F.L.. Mercury from dental "silver" tooth fillings impairs sheep kidney function. American Journal of Physiology. 261:R1010-R1014, 1991.

[3] Summers, A.O., Wireman, J., Vimy, M.J., Lorscheider, F.L., Marshal, B., Levy, S.B., Bennet, S., Billard, L.. Journal of Anti-Microbial Agents and Chemotherapy. 37(4):825-834, April 1993.

# Other Sources of Information

Interstitial Cystitis Association (ICA)
51 Monroe Street
Suite #1402
Rockville, MD  20850
Phone: (301) 610-5308
Fax: (301) 610-5300

Cystitis Research Center
4021 Wonderland Drive
Rapid City, South Dakota  57702
Phone: (605) 342-8989
Fax: (605) 342-8989

Interstitial Cystitis Information Center (ICIC)
1706 Briery Road
Farmville, Virginia  23901
Kay Benton, Director

American Pain Society
5700 Old Orchard Road
Skokie, IL  60077
Phone: (708) 966-5595

American Uro-Gynecologic Society
401 North Michigan Avenue
Chicago, IL  60611-4267
Phone: (312) 644-6610

International Pain Foundation
909 Northeast 43rd Street, Suite 306
Seattle, WA  98105-6020
Phone: (206) 547-2157

National Kidney and Urologic Diseases Information Clearinghouse
3 Information Way
Bethesda, MD 20892-3580
Phone: (301) 654-4415

National Organization of Social Security Claimants' Representatives
6 Prospect Street
Midland Park, NJ 07432
Phone: 1-800-431-2804

The British Columbia Interstitial Cystitis Association
#1204--2024 Fullerton Avenue
North Vancouver, BC
Canada V7P 3G4
Phone: (604) 922-1407
Fax: (604) 931-6293

Canadian Interstitial Cystitis Society (CICS)
PO Box 28625
Burnaby, BC Canada
V5C 6J4
Phone: (250) 758-3207

1-888-ELMIRON

Biotel Corp
366 Madison Avenue #1506
New York, NY 10017
Phone: 1-800-445-4551
(to purchase home urine tests)

The Vulvar Pain Foundation
Post Office Drawer 177
Graham, North Carolina 27253
Phone: (336) 226-0704
Fax: (336) 226-8518

Sjogren's Syndrome Foundation
333 North Broadway
Jericho, New York  11753
Phone: 1-800-4-SJOGRENS

The CFIDS Association, Inc.
PO Box 220398
Charlotte, NC  28222
Phone: 1-800-442-3437

Lupus Foundation of America
4 Research Place, Suite #180
Rockville, MD  20850
Phone: 1-800-558-0121

Fibromyalgia Network
5800 Stockdale Highway #100
Bakersfield, CA  93309
Phone: (805) 631-1950

Endometriosis Association
8585 N. 76th Place
Milwaukee, WI  53223
Phone: 1-800-992-3636

Raynaud's Foundation
P.O. Box 346176
Chicago, IL  60634-6176
Phone: (773) 622-9220
Fax: (773) 622-9221

The Pain Clinic (Dr. Devi Nambudripad)
6714 Beach Blvd.
Buena Park, CA  90621
Phone: (714) 523-0800

# Exploring IC Through the Internet

If you don't have a computer at home, you can go to most libraries these days and use one there. There is a huge amount of information available about IC on the net that is well worth checking out. Be a well informed patient and speak to other IC patients and read the current research and treatment trends. The following are a list of Internet addresses to get you started. As you probably know, Internet addresses change frequently. These were current as of January 1998. You can also do a search on Interstitial Cystitis on one of the many search engines available, such as Yahoo, Google, Hotbot, etc.

IC Hope for Interstitial Cystitis
http://www.ic-hope.com

Interstitial Cystitis Association (ICA)
http://www.ichelp.org

Interstitial Cystitis Information Center
http://www.moonstar.com/~icickay

Intercyst
http://www.intercyst.org

NIDDK
http://www.niddk.nih.gov/InterstitialCystitis/InterstitialCystitis.html

Interstitial Cystitis "An Herbal Approach"
http://chili.rt66.com:80/hrbmoore/ManualsMM/ISCHerbs.txt

Cystitis Research Center
http://pw1.netcom.com/~jewel3/uti/bacteria.html

The Prostatitis Foundation
http://prostate.org

FDA Page on IC
http://www.fda.gov:80/fdac/features/995_cystitis.html

Redbook IC article
http://homearts.com/rb/health/05infeb4.htm

MedAccess IC article
http://www.medaccess.com:80/consumer_rep/hc0100.htm

Medscape
http://www.medscape.com

Reuters Health News
http://reutershealth.com

Pharmaceutical Information Network
http:/www.pharminfo.com

NORD - NIH/National Kidney and Urologic
http://www.stepstn.com:80/nord/rdb_sum/103.htm

The National Sjogren's Syndrome Association (has a page on IC)
http://www.sjogrens.org

The Vulvar Pain Foundation
http://www.vulvarpainfoundation.org/index.html

Raynaud's Foundation
http://members.aol.com/raynauds/index.htm

N.A.E.T. - Nampudripad Allergy Elimination Technique
http://www.naet.com

# Appendix

## Presenting The America On Line
### INTERSTITIAL CYSTITIS PATIENT RESEARCH
### QUESTIONNAIRE
## Results - May 1997

In sincere appreciation for those with Interstitial Cystitis who participated in this questionnaire. Those who with determination and compassion took the time to become involved in the search for a cure. I appreciate your honesty and uncompromising sincerity.

Bravely and with hope in our hearts we reach for the hand of God . . . .
Suzanne Bernhardt

01. WHAT IS YOUR CURRENT AGE?
The youngest person is 20. The oldest person is 76. The median age is 44.

02. WHAT IS YOUR ON-LINE NAME?
03. WHAT IS YOUR FIRST NAME?
See credits last page.

04. WHAT STATE DO YOU LIVE IN?
Respondents were from all across the US and Canada. The states most often mentioned are listed in order of frequency: California, Georgia, Illinois and New York.

05. HOW LONG HAVE YOU HAD BLADDER TROUBLE OF ANY KIND?
An enormous variation in years ranging from 1.5 years to 50 years with a median of 17.5 years.

06. HOW LONG HAVE YOU BEEN DIAGNOSED WITH IC?
A range of 2 months to 19 years with a median of 4.2 years.

07. WHAT DO YOU THINK IS THE NUMBER ONE CAUSE OF YOUR IC?
I believe all of the theories are important so listed here in order are all of the answers received.

Don't Know 17%
Bacteria 15%
Surgery/Catheter 15%

Dysfunctional Immune System 11%
Stress 9%
Hereditary Factor (from birth) 7%
Recurrent Bladder Infections 6%
Hysterectomy 4%
Neurological 3%
Leaking Breast Implants 1.0%
Virus in the Nerves 1.0%
Vulvodynia 1.0%
Poor Health 1.0%
Food Allergies 1.0%
Repressed Anger 1.0%
Sacral Nerve Malfunction 1.0%
Water 1.0%
Herniated Disk 1.0%
Unidentified Substance in the Urine 1.0%
Untreated Kidney Infection 1.0%
Defective or Damaged Bladder 1.0%
Overuse of Antibiotics 1.0%


## 08. WHAT DO YOU THINK IS THE NUMBER TWO CAUSE OF YOUR IC?

I believe all of the theories are important so listed here in order are all of the answers received.

Don't Know 26%
Dysfunctional Immune System 13%
Bacteria 8%
Stress 7%
Hormones 5%
Surgery/Catheter 5%
Hereditary 5%
Bladder Damaged from Multi Infections/Antibiotics 4%
Allergies 4%
Spinal 4%
Hysterectomy 3%
Endometriosis 3%
Sexually transmitted Disease 3%
Acidity 3%
Overuse of Antibiotics 1%
Recreational Drugs 1%
Sexual Abuse 1%

Cystoscope 1%
Herniated Disk 1%
Bladder irritants 1%
DMSO 1%

## 09. HAS YOUR IC GOTTEN WORSE OVER TIME - DEGENERATIVE?
50% said Yes
50% said No

## 10. DO YOU HAVE ENDOMETRIOSIS?
72% said No
20% said Yes
8% said Don't Know

## 11. HAVE YOU EVER BEEN TOLD YOU HAVE TRIGONITIS?
89% said No
10% said Yes
1% said Not Applicable

## 12. WHAT OTHER DISEASES OR HEALTH PROBLEMS DO YOU HAVE IN ADDITION TO IC ?
The answers to this questions were way too numerous to list so noted here are the most mentioned.

IBS 29%                              (key: % = of participants)
Fibromyalgia 18%
Allergies/Sinus 18%
Migraines 18%
No Other Diseases 15%
Back Problems 11%
Vulvodynia 10%
Hypothyroidism 8%
Mitral Valve Prolapse 8%
High Blood Pressure 6%
Arthritis 6%
Achy Joints 4%
Endometriosis 4%
Yeast 4%
Hypoglycemia 3%

## 13. DO YOU THINK THAT IC HAS SOMETHING TO DO WITH YOUR IMMUNE SYSTEM?

72% said Yes
15% said No
13% said Don't know

## 14. IF YES, SPECIFICALLY HOW HAS IC AFFECTED YOUR IMMUNE SYSTEM?

52% said IC Lowered Their Immune System.
27% said Not Applicable.
13% said Their Immune System Caused The IC
7% said Don't Know
1% said Other

## 15. DID YOU WET YOUR BED WHEN YOU WERE YOUNG?

75% said No
22% said Yes
3% said Don't Know

## 16. WHAT AGE WERE WHEN YOU STOPPED WETTING THE BED?

Among those that answered Yes to #15 answered ranged from age 3 to age 18 with a median of 8.

## 17. DID YOU EVER HOLD YOUR URINE FOR LONG PERIODS AT A TIME WHEN YOU WERE YOUNG STALLING GOING TO THE BATHROOM FOR WHAT EVER REASON?

53% said Yes.
37% said No
6% said Not Applicable
4% said Don't Know

## 18. DO YOU THINK STRESS IS THE CAUSE OF IC?

72% said No
20% said Yes
8% said Don't Know

## 19. DO YOU THINK STRESS AFFECTS YOUR IC?

92% said Yes
7% said No
1% said Not Applicable

## 20. BRIEFLY HOW DOES STRESS AFFECT YOUR IC?

60% said Stress Increases All Symptoms
13% said Stress Causes flare-ups and muscle spasms
10% said Not Applicable
6% said  Stress Weakens the Immune System
6% said  Other
3% said  Stress hurts the entire body
1% said  Stress causes increased body acidity
1% said  Stress increases frequency

## 21. WHAT TYPE OF STRESS AFFECTS YOUR IC (WORK, NERVOUSNESS, WORRY, ETC)?

63% said Worry/Anxiety          (key: % = of participants)
20% said Any or All Stress
17% said Work
8% said Not Applicable
8% said Anger
6% said Sleeplessness
3% said Fear
1% said Don't Know
1% said Physical Activity

## 22. WHAT DO YOU DO TO COMBAT STRESS EFFECTIVELY?

All answers are listed here in order of most frequently said.
Relaxation
Exercise
Meditation
Detachment
Deep Breathing
Listen to Music/Sing
Prayer
Take a Hot Bath
Read
Talk to People
Yoga
Therapy
Gardening
Humor
Light Candles
Self Hypnosis
Diet
Aromatherapy

## 23. DO YOU THINK THAT IC IS BACTERIALLY RELATED?
65% said Yes
21% said Don't Know
14% said No


## 24. WHY DO YOU THINK IC IS BACTERIALLY RELATED?
26 % said Not Applicable
17 % said They Have Gotten A Positive Reaction From Antibiotics
11 % said Dr. Fugazotto Found Bacteria In Their Urine
10 % said They Have Had Many Positive Urine Cultures
10 % said Don't Know
5   % said Bacteria Is How Their IC Started
3   % said IC Acts Like A Disease Process
3   % said  There is An Overabundance of Resident Bacteria
3   % said IC Feels Like A Bladder Infection
3   % said They Got IC From Surgery
3   % said It Makes Sense
3   % said Bacteria is The Cause Of Constant Inflammation
1   % said  IC is Transmitted through sex
1   % said IC is Transmitted Through Improper Hygiene
1   % said The IC Immune System Allows Bacteria to Multiply


## 25. DO YOU THINK YOUR SEX PARTNER CONTRIBUTES TO A BACTERIAL PROBLEM?
45% said No
31% said Yes
13% said Not Applicable
11% said Don't Know


## 26. DID YOUR IC BEGIN AS THE RESULT OF SURGERY OR A PROCEDURE IN THE HOSPITAL?
56% said No
32% said Yes
8% said Possibly
4% Don't Know


## 27. DO YOU THINK YOUR IC IS RELATED TO A STAPH INFECTION OR BACTERIA?
39% said Yes
28% said No
20% said Don't Know
13% said Maybe

## 28. WHY DO YOU THINK IC IS RELATED TO A STAPH INFECTION OR BACTERIA?

37% said Not Applicable
13% said Don't Know
11% said They Have Had Many Positive Urine Cultures
8% said Dr. Fugazotto Found Bacteria In Their Urine
8% said It Seems Logical
7% said They Got IC From Surgery
4% said IC is Like A Stomach Ulcer and that is Bacteria
3% said The IC Symptoms Point To Bacteria
3% said That's How Their IC Started
3% said They Have Had Positive Reactions To Antibiotics
1% said They Had Many Yeast infections
1% said They had A Staph Infection At Birth
1% said Bacteria is Attacking The Bladder Wall

## 29. HAVE YOU BEEN ON DR. FUGAZZOTTO'S TREATMENT?

82% said No
18% said Yes

## 30. ARE YOU CURRENTLY UNDERGOING DR. FUGAZZOTTO'S TREATMENT?

77% said No
13% said Not Applicable
10% said Yes

## 31. IS OR DID DR. FUGAZZOTTO'S TREATMENT WORK FOR YOU?

80% said Not Applicable
14% said Yes
6% said No

## 32. IF DR. FUGAZZOTTO'S TREATMENT DID NOT WORK FOR YOU WHY NOT?

Of The 6% Who Answered No to #31 Their Answers Follow:
Antibiotics Were Too Painful
Yeast Was a Big Problem
Long Term Antibiotics Are Too Dangerous To The Body

## 33. DOES ANYONE ELSE IN YOUR FAMILY OR FAMILY TREE HAVE IC?

85% said No
9% said Yes
4% said Don't Know

## 34. WHAT RELATIONSHIP IN YOUR FAMILY OR FAMILY TREE ALSO HAS OR HAD IC?

Of the 7% Who Answered Yes to #33 Their Answers Follow in order of Most Frequently Answered :
Sister
Mother
Daughter
Cousin
Niece

## 35. DOES ANYONE ELSE IN YOUR FAMILY OR FAMILY TREE HAVE BLADDER PROBLEMS (LIKE INFECTIONS BUT NOT IC)?

46% said Yes
45% said No
9% said Don't Know

## 36. WHAT RELATIONSHIP IN YOUR FAMILY OR FAMILY TREE HAS OR HAD BLADDER PROBLEMS BUT WAS NOT DIAGNOSED WITH IC?

Of the 46% That Answered Yes To #35 Their Answers Follow in order of Most Frequently Answered :
Mother
Sister
Grandmother
Aunt
Daughter
Cousin
Granddaughter
Father
Brother
Uncle
Niece

## 37. HAS YOUR HUSBAND OR SEX PARTNER EVER HAD A BLADDER INFECTION?

79% said No
11% said Yes
10% said Not Applicable

## 38. DID YOU LIVE IN AN AREA GROWING UP THAT WAS SPRAYED WITH PESTICIDES REGULARLY?

56% said No
31% said Yes
13% said Don't Know

## 39. DID YOU LIVE ON A MILITARY BASE GROWING UP?
86% said No
14% said Yes

## 40. IF NOT A MILITARY BASE WHERE DID YOU LIVE AROUND PESTICIDES?
70% said Not Applicable
Of the Other 30% 2/3 lived in cities or towns, 1/3 lived on or near farms

## 41. WHAT WERE THE PESTICIDES USED FOR?
General Bug Killing and/or Crop Dusting

## 42. DO YOU KNOW WHAT SPECIFIC PESTICIDES THEY WERE?
99% replied No or Not Applicable
1% said DDT

## 43. DO YOU USE A HOME WATER FILTER?
52% said No
48% said Yes or Use Bottled Water

## 44. HAVE YOU EVER CONSIDERED YOUR IC PROBLEMS TO HAVE ANYTHING TO DO WITH YOUR WATER?
69% said No
31% said Yes

## 45. HAVE YOU HAD YOUR WATER TESTED?
82% said No
18% said Yes

## 46. IF YES, WHAT WERE THE RESULTS OF YOUR WATER TESTING?
82% said Not Applicable
10% said It Was OK
3% said It tested Positive For Iron
3% said It Tested Positive For Large Amounts Of Pollutants
2% said It Tested Positive For Chlorine

## 47. PLEASE LIST WHAT DRUGS EFFECT YOUR IC POSITIVELY
Over 100 Different Drugs Were Mentioned. Listed Here **IN ORDER** are the Most Frequently Answered:
**Peridium**
**Antibiotics**

Elmiron
Elavil
None
Ibuprofen
DMSO
Urised
Ditropan
Demerol
Heparin
Noroxin
Valium
Levbid
Alive
Antihistamines
Ultram
Vistaril
Kenalog
Levsin
Levinex
Prozac
Klonopin

## 48. PLEASE LIST WHAT DRUGS EFFECT YOUR IC NEGATIVELY.

Too many to list. Mentioned here **IN ORDER** of importance are all answers that got more than one mention.
None
Some Antibiotics
DMSO
Antihistamines
Elavil
Chlorpactin
Elmiron
Cortisone
Antidepressants

## 49. PLEASE LIST WHAT TREATMENTS (OTHER THAN DRUGS) THAT EFFECT YOUR IC POSITIVELY.

Answers Listed in Order of Frequency:
None!
Hot Bath/Hot Water bottle/Heating Pad
Diet

Hydrodistension
Drinking Lots of Water
Rest & Relaxation
Colloidal Minerals
Exercise
Bladder Installations
Massage Therapy
All of the following got one response each:
Physical therapy
Vacation
Bladder Dilation
Herbs
Psychic Healer
Tens Unit
Acupressure
Meditation
Bladder Training
DMSO
RIMSO
Dr. Whitmore Bladder Installation Cocktail


## 50. PLEASE LIST WHAT TREATMENTS (OTHER THAN DRUGS) THAT EFFECT YOUR IC NEGATIVELY

Answers Listed in Order of Frequency:
None
Hydrodistension
Invasive Bladder Installations
Diet
Cystoscope
Gillespie Bladder Installation Cocktail
Cranberry
Sex


## 51. PLEASE LIST ANY VITAMINS OR HERBS THAT HAVE EFFECTED YOUR IC POSITIVELY.

Answers Listed in Order of Frequency of Mention:
None Or Not Applicable
Antioxidants (E,A,D)
Marshmallow Root
Buffered or Ester C
L-Arginine
Herbal Teas

Acidopholis
Garlic
Echinacea
Vitamins
Trace Colloidal Minerals
Goldenseal
Siberian Ginseng
Aloe Vera
Magnesium
Zinc
Evening Primrose
Calcium
Ginko Biloba
The following were mentioned one time each: Multi Vitamins, Bypassand
Rejuvacel, Usana, Silver, Uva ursi, Grapeseed Extract, Adrenal
Supplements, Croned tarr, Calcium Citrate, N Acetyl Glucosamine,
Dandelion Root, Cornsilk, Valerian Root, Parsley, Bee Pollen, Amino
Acids, URY & SBK, Ginger, Spirulina, Selenium, Yeast Fighters, Cat's
Claw, Comfrey Root, B6, White Willow Bark.

## 52. PLEASE LIST ANY VITAMINS OR HERBS THAT HAVE EFFECTED YOUR IC NEGATIVELY.

Answers Listed in Order of Frequency of Mention:
None, Not applicable or Don't Know
Unbuffered Vitamin C
Vitamin B
Multi Vitamins
Citric Tea, IC Tea, Catnip Tea, Chinese Herbal Tea, Pao Tea
The following were mentioned one time each:
Diet Suppressants, Cranberry, Amino Acids, Astragalus, Citric Acid,
DHEA, Too Much goldenseal, Too much Echinacea, Acidolpholis,
Calcium, Everything, DHR for Migraines.

## 53. HAVE YOU EVER BEEN TOLD THAT YOU HAVE A CYST IN YOUR KIDNEYS?

96% said No
4% said Yes

## 54. HAVE YOU EVER BEEN TOLD THAT YOU HAVE KIDNEY STONES?

87% said No
10% said Yes
3% said Maybe

## 55. HAVE YOU EVER HAD ANY OTHER KIDNEY PROBLEMS?
76% said No
24% said Yes

## 56. WHAT KIDNEY PROBLEM DID YOU HAVE?
Of the 24% That Answered Yes to #55 The Following Were Their Answers
In Order Of Frequency:
Kidney Infections
Kidney Stones
Buildup Blocking Path From Kidneys
Blocked Ureter
Kidney Reflux
Abnormal Shape
Pyelonephritis

## 57. DOES OR DID ANYONE IN YOUR FAMILY OR FAMILY TREE HAVE KIDNEY PROBLEMS?
63% said No
34% said Yes
3% said Don't Know

## 58. WHAT KIND OF KIDNEY PROBLEMS DID YOUR FAMILY MEMBER HAVE?
Of the 34% Who Answered Yes to #57 The Following Are Their Answers
In Order Of Frequency:
Kidney Stones
Kidney Infection
Nephritis
Kidney Replacement
Kidney Failure
Uremic Poisoning

## 59. WHAT RELATION WERE THEY TO YOU?
Of the 34% Who Answered Yes to #57 The Following Are Their Answers
In Order Of Frequency:
Father
Mother
Cousin
Sister
Husband
Grandmother
Great Grandmother
Brother
Niece

## 60. DO YOU CONSUME FIBER REGULARLY?
70% said Yes
30% said No

## 61. WHAT SOURCE(S) OF FIBER DO YOU USE REGULARLY OR MOST OFTEN?
Answers Listed in Order Of frequency:
Vegetables/Salads
Cereal
Bread/Grains
None
Fruit (Prunes, Raisins, Pears, Apples and Others)
Beans
Metamucil
Psyllium Husks
Fibercon/Fiberall
Mentioned Once Each: Citricel, Fiber bars, Slimfast, Pasta, Herbal Laxative, Nuts

## 62. DO YOU HAVE AT LEAST ONE BOWEL MOVEMENT A DAY?
79% said Yes
18% said No
3% said Sometimes

## 63. DO YOU HAVE IRRITABLE BOWEL SYNDROME ?
51% said No
49% said Yes

## 64. DO YOU HAVE HIGH BLOOD PRESSURE?
85% said No
15% said Yes

## 65. HAVE YOU EVER HAD THE PH OF YOUR URINE TESTED?
51% said No
45% said Yes
4% Don't Know

## 66. THROUGH THE TEST WAS YOUR URINE MORE ALKALINE OR ACIDIC?
52% said Not Applicable
17% said Don't Know
17% said Alkaline
14% said Acidic

## 67. DO YOU HAVE EXCESSIVE GAS?
52% said No
35% said Yes
13% said Sometimes

## 68. DO YOU THINK HORMONES PLAY A PART IN IC?
55% said Yes
24% said No
14% said Don't know
7% said Maybe

## 69. IF YES, WHY DO YOU THINK HORMONES EFFECT IC?
Answers Listed in Order Of frequency:
Pain fluctuates with period and ovulation
Many women with IC have other female related problems
Hormones, the Immune System and IC are all related
Uneven hormone levels affect blood chemistry
Estrogen replacement therapy helps IC
IC pain fluctuates with pregnancy
IC pain fluctuates with menopause
Hormones are effected by infections

## 70. DOES YOUR IC FLARE UP RIGHT BEFORE YOUR PERIOD?
51% said Yes
39% said Not Applicable
10% said No

## 71. IS YOUR IC BETTER DURING YOUR PERIOD?
46% said Not Applicable
31% said Yes
23% said No

## 72. DOES YOUR IC FLARE UP RIGHT AFTER YOUR PERIOD?
44% said Not Applicable
38% said No
17% said Yes
1% said Don't Know

## 73. DOES YOU IC FLARE UP TWO WEEKS AFTER YOUR PERIOD?
48% said Not Applicable
31% said Yes
21% said No

## 74. HAVE YOU EVER TAKEN BIRTH CONTROL PILLS AS A TREATMENT FOR IC?

77% said No
15% said Yes
8% said No

## 75. IF YOU TOOK BIRTH CONTROL PILLS FOR IC - DID THEY HELP YOUR IC SYMPTOMS?

77% said Not Applicable
13% said No
10% said Yes

## 76. ARE YOU COLD A LOT OF THE TIME?

68% said Yes
29% said No
3% said Sometimes

## 77. ARE YOU HOT A LOT OF THE TIME?

63% said No
30% said Yes
7% said Sometimes

## 78. PLEASE LIST THE FOLLOWING IN THE ORDER OF WHAT BEST HELPS YOUR IC SYMPTOMS? HERBS? ORAL DRUGS? BLADDER INSTALLATIONS? RELAXATION? OTHER CATEGORY?

50% listed Oral Drugs as their **NUMBER ONE** choice to help IC symptoms
14% listed Bladder Installations as their **NUMBER ONE** choice to help IC symptoms
10% listed Other (see below) as their **NUMBER ONE** choice to help IC symptoms
10% listed Relaxation as their **NUMBER ONE** choice to help IC symptoms
8% listed no first choice as their **NUMBER ONE** choice to help IC symptoms
7% listed Diet as their **NUMBER ONE** choice to help IC symptoms
1% listed Bladder Distension as their **NUMBER ONE** choice to help IC symptoms

31% listed No Second Choice as their **NUMBER TWO** choice to help IC symptoms
24% listed Relaxation as their **NUMBER TWO** choice to help IC symptoms

212

14% listed Oral Drugs as their **NUMBER TWO** choice to help IC symptoms

10% listed Other (see below) as their **NUMBER TWO** choice to help IC symptoms

9% listed Diet as their **NUMBER TWO** choice to help IC symptoms

7% listed Bladder Installations as their **NUMBER TWO** choice to help IC symptoms

4% listed Herbs as their **NUMBER TWO** choice to help IC symptoms

1% listed Bladder Installations as their **NUMBER TWO** choice to help IC symptoms


54% listed No Third Choice as their **NUMBER THREE** choice to help IC symptoms

12% listed Herbs as their **NUMBER THREE** choice to help IC symptoms

10% listed Relaxation as their **NUMBER THREE** choice to help IC symptoms

8% listed Oral Drugs as their **NUMBER THREE** choice to help IC symptoms

7% listed Other (see below) as their **NUMBER THREE** choice to help IC symptoms

4% listed Diet as their **NUMBER THREE** choice to help IC symptoms

3% listed Exercise as their **NUMBER THREE** choice to help IC symptoms

1% listed Bladder Distension as their **NUMBER THREE** choice to help IC symptoms

1% listed Bladder Installations as their **NUMBER THREE** choice to help IC symptoms


70% listed No Fourth Choice as their **NUMBER FOUR** choice to help IC symptoms

8% listed Other (see below) as their **NUMBER FOUR** choice to help IC symptoms

8% listed Herbs as their **NUMBER FOUR** choice to help IC symptoms

7% listed Relaxation as their **NUMBER FOUR** choice to help IC symptoms

4% listed Bladder Installations as their **NUMBER FOUR** choice to help IC symptoms

3% listed Diet as their **NUMBER FOUR** choice to help IC symptoms


**OTHER** choices were: Hot Baths, Minerals, Physical Therapy, Holistic Treatments, Personal Regime, Drink Water, Nerve Stimulator, Baking Soda, Tums, Tens Unit, Chiropractor, Acupuncture, Meditation, Stress Reduction, Yoga and Psychic Healer.

## 79. DO YOU HAVE ALLERGIES OF ANY KIND?
70% said Yes
28% said No
2% said Don't Know

## 80. DO YOU HAVE ALLERGIES TO FOOD?
63% said No
30% said Yes
7% said Don't Know

## 81. DO YOU HAVE ALLERGIES TO PLANTS OR MOLDS?
50% said No
44% said Yes
6% said Don't Know

## 82. IF YOU KNOW EXACTLY WHAT YOU ARE ALLERGIC TO PLEASE LIST:
Here again a wide variety of substances too numerous to list. Listed here are the things that received more than one response in order of frequency.
**Mildew/Mold Fungus**
**Grasses/Trees/Pollen**
Animals, Dust/Mites, Sulfa, Dairy, Metal, Chemical Cleaners, Feathers, Egg Whites, Fragrances, Shell Fish

## 83. CAN YOU TAKE ANTIHISTAMINES?
69% said Yes
28% said No
2% said Don't Know
1% said Not Applicable

## 84. DO ANTIHISTAMINES HELP OR HURT YOUR IC SYMPTOMS?
52% said Not Applicable
28% said They Hurt IC Symptoms
9% said They Help IC Symptoms
8% said Don't Know
3% said They Don't Hurt IC Symptoms

## 85. DID PREGNANCY POSITIVELY OR NEGATIVELY EFFECT YOUR IC?
80% said Not Applicable
10% said Pregnancy had a Positive Effect On Their IC
6% said Don't Know
4% said Pregnancy has a Negative Effect on Their IC

214

86. DID YOU TAKE DRUGS FOR IC DURING YOUR PREGNANCY?
73% said Not Applicable
23% said No
4% said Yes

87. IF YOU TOOK IC DRUGS DURING YOUR PREGNANCY WHAT DID YOU TAKE?
Elavil
Peridium
Seconal
Pain Medications and Antibiotics

88. DID YOU HAVE ANY PROBLEMS OR COMPLICATIONS DURING PREGNANCY THAT YOU THINK MAY HAVE BEEN RELATED TO YOUR IC OR ANY IC DRUGS YOU TOOK WHILE PREGNANT?
96% said Not Applicable
4% said Yes

89. IF YES, WHAT PROBLEMS WITH PREGNANCY RELATED TO IC DID YOU EXPERIENCE?
1. Had terrible case of Laguna Lakes. Placenta was destroyed at Birth and was sent to lab for autopsy. Patient took Elavil for entire pregnancy. Fetus was perfectly healthy although she held her urine longer than normal in vitro.
2. Unusual pain and frequency
3. Gestational Diabetes
4. Had to have catheter during labor to void
5. Kidney function problems while pregnant only
6. Miscarried while on Nortriphine

90. DO YOU THINK IC HAS ANY THING TO DO WITH THYROID PROBLEMS OR VICE VERSA?
45% said No
35% said Don't Know
14% said Maybe
6% said Yes

91. IF YES, HOW DO YOU THINK IC IS RELATED TO THYROID PROBLEMS OR VICE VERSA?
1. Thyroid created a hormonal imbalance which opened the door to IC.
2. Thyroid function is lowered because of constant infection.
3. It's an auto immune disease.
4. The body is out of balance.

5. I may have been wrongly diagnosed and treated for thyroid problems.
6. My hormone levels keep changing.
7. I have both diseases.
8. IC infection is systemic - it travels through the blood, emitting toxins and poisons effecting various organs - mostly the weakest. Bladder and Thyroid included.

## 92. DO YOU THINK IC HAS ANYTHING TO DO WITH DIABETES OR VICE VERSA?
51% said No
31% said Don't Know
7% said Yes
7% said Maybe
4% said Not Applicable

## 93. IF YES, HOW DO YOU THINK IC IS RELATED TO DIABETES OR VICE VERSA?
1. Diabetes is created from constant infections
2. My mother has diabetes.
3. The body is out of balance
4. Its an auto immune disease
5. Compromised immune system
6. Diabetes is related to blood sugar and IC travels through the blood.

## 94. ARE YOU OFTEN BLOATED?
72% said Yes
28% said No

## 95. ARE YOU OFTEN CONSTIPATED?
62% said Yes
38% said No

## 96. DO YOU FEEL BETTER AFTER A LARGE OR COMPLETE BOWEL MOVEMENT OR CLEANSING?
79% said Yes
15% said No
6% said Not Applicable

## 97. DO YOU FEEL WORSE WHEN YOU ARE BLOATED AND CONSTIPATED?
86% said Yes
7% said Not Applicable
4% said No
3% said Not Sure

## 98. DO YOU EXERCISE?
81% said Yes
18% said No
1% said Rarely

## 99. WHAT TYPE OF EXERCISE DO YOU DO?
All answers are listed here in order of frequency of mention:
Walking
Not Applicable
Weights
Low Impact Aerobics/Water Aerobics
Volley Ball/Tennis/Racket Ball
Biking
Stretching
Treadmill
Yoga
Running
Swimming
Nautilus
Nordic Track
Sit-Ups
Gardening
Dancing
Housework
The following got one answer each: Pelvic Floor Exercise, Horse Riding, Rollerblading, Cardio, Stairmaster, Health Rider

## 100. WITH WHAT REGULARITY DO YOU EXERCISE?
27% said 3 X week
17% said 2 X week
15% said Daily
14% said Never
10% said 1 X week
6% said 5 X week
4% said 4 X week
4% said 6 X week
3% said Not applicable

## 101. DO YOU THINK EXERCISE HELPS YOUR IC?
61% said Yes
22% said No
11% said Not Applicable
6% said Don't Know

## 102. WHY DO YOU THINK EXERCISE HELPS YOUR IC?

Exercise Increases blood circulation
Exercise creates a positive chemical reaction
Exercise increases muscle tone
Exercise stretches and tones the body
Exercise relieves stress
Exercise is relaxing
Exercise stimulates the bowels
Exercise promotes mental and physical strengthening
Exercise improves general health
Exercise gives control over IC
Exercise increases energy levels
Exercise is a good distraction
Exercise increases endorphins
Exercise stimulates the mind, spirit and body
Exercise makes you feel better.
Exercise keeps me sane
Exercise flushes out toxins

## 103. IF YOU THINK EXERCISE HURTS YOUR IC PLEASE EXPLAIN.

Sometimes it hurts when I exercise but I always feel better afterwards.
Sweating in the groin area makes me feel worse.
Sometimes I have pain afterward in the Urethra
Sometimes it increases the pain of IC
Aerobics or excessive jumping cause pain to be worse
Cannot exercise during flareups
It hurts to contract pelvic muscles
Too much exercise hurts my bladder

## 104. DO YOU DRINK A LOT OF WATER?

70% said Yes
23% said No
7% said Average

## 105. HOW MANY GLASSES OF WATER DO YOU DRINK DURING THE DAY?

45% said they drink 0 - 5 glasses of water a day
34% said they drink 6 - 9 glasses of water a day
21% said they drink more than 10 glasses of water a day

## 106. WHAT IS THE NUMBER ONE SOURCE OF LIQUID YOU DRINK DURING THE DAY?
89% said Water
4% said Soda/Diet Soda
3% said Coffee
3% said Milk
1% said Sports Drink

## 107. WHAT IS THE NUMBER TWO SOURCE OF LIQUID YOU DRINK DURING THE DAY?
23% said Water
21% said Herbal/Decaf Tea
14% said Milk
12% said Soda
11% said Juice
10% said Coffee
8% said Nothing
1% said Koolaid

## 108. HOW MANY CUPS OF COFFEE DO YOU DRINK DURING THE DAY?
49% said Zero
25% said One
11% said Two
6% said Three
6% said 1/2 cup
3% said More than three cups

## 109. NAME ONE TO THREE FOODS THAT IF YOU EAT WILL DEFINITELY NEGATIVELY AFFECT YOUR IC.
The most frequently mentioned foods listed here in order of importance:
**Juices/Citrus Fruits/Acidic Fruits**
**Tomatoes/Acidic Foods**
**Spicy Sauces/Spicy Foods**
Soda
Coffee
Lemonade
Vinegar/Salad Dressings
Chocolate
No negative food affects
Alcohol
Nutrasweet

Apples
Bananas
Onions
Sugar
Tea
Caffeine
Milk
Hot Dogs/ Salami/Pepperoni
The following were mentioned once each: Soy Sauce, Theater popcorn,
Slimfast, Garlic, Peppers, Walnuts, Marinades, Preservatives, MSG,
Asparagus, grapes

## 110. NAME ANY FOOD(S) THAT HAVE A POSITIVE AFFECT ON YOUR IC. (IN OTHER WORDS A FOOD THAT ACTUALLY HELPS YOUR SYMPTOMS PLEASE DO NOT LIST ALL THE FOODS YOU CAN EAT).

None
Baking Soda
Tums
Pasta/Breads/Rice
Green Vegetables
Yellow Vegetables
Potatoes
Milk
Carbohydrates
Tea (esp. Chamomile)
The following were mentioned once each: Grapes, Meat, Cheese, Pears,
Cheeseburgers, Molasses, Garlic, Soda crackers.

## 111. ARE THERE ANY OTHER THINGS (OTHER THAN LISTED HERE) THAT YOU THINK COULD HAVE CAUSED YOUR IC?

65% said No

Neurological
Spiritual Pain
Pesticides
Hysterectomy
Endometriosis
Viral Causes
Epstein Barr Virus
Missed Diagnosis
Over prescribed antibiotics
Sex may exacerbate an underlying condition

Other answers:

Spinal Cord Alignment
Vaginal Infections
Bacterial Cystitis
Previous Surgeries
Sexually transmitted disease
Hereditary
Not enough studies done on men with
    IC
Vaginal Imbalance

## 112. HAVE I TOUCHED ON THEORIES YOU HAVE HAD?
83% said Yes
14% said No
3% said Don't Know

## 113. DO YOU HAVE ANY OTHER THEORIES OR ISSUES OF CONCERN?
Note: About half of the participants had an answer to this question. I believe that concerns and opinions of actual IC patients are very viable to finding a cure. Listed below are ALL the answers to this question:

1. What puts people in remission?
2. What is the involvement of bacteria/pathogens?
3. What is the connection between a slipped disk, foot pain and IC?
4. Is IC infection that never went away?
5. Is IC a result of an antibiotic treatment?
6. Is IC an auto immune reaction triggered by infection?
7. Is IC nerve, tissue or muscle damage caused by infection?
8. What is the relativity of sex and its connection to the cause or perpetuation of IC?
9. Most Urologists are uneducated about IC and continue with the medieval and expensive invasive
   treatments. Are researchers looking into the bacterial connection?
10. How is IC related to the bowels, ovaries, uterus, lower back and sinuses?
11. Why hasn't the antibiotic theory been more aggressively pursued by the medical community?
12. Is the bladder being damaged during pelvic surgery making it susceptible to IC?
13. Why is the odor of IC patient's urine so strong?
14. If the disease's pain is caused by ulcerations/tears/irritation to the bladder wall, then why can't a researcher isolate something foreign in IC afflicted patients that is not present in non-IC patients?
15. Is there a heretical connection?
16. Is this disease being swept under the carpet because the vast majority of IC patients are women?
17. Why isn't Dr. Fugazzotto's treatment plan for IC being given more credence?
18. What connection is there if any between IC and neurological disorders? There should be further study on the nerves in the brain that control the bladder, colon, uterus and pelvic organs.
19. There needs to be more research on the auto immune disease connection - vulvodynia, IBS, Fibromyalgia, CFS and burning tongue and mouth are all related.

20. There needs to be more research on treating the body, mind and spirit as one - as in Middle Eastern Philosophy.

21. Why is the medical community so slow in figuring out this disease?

22. Chemotherapy for breast cancer helped my IC along with antibiotics what is the connection?

23. Why are doctors (including Urologists) so uninformed about IC?

24. How after six months of being on Elmiron can one get a bladder infection? (It happened)

25. How can just one UTI turn into IC? What is the connection between IC and edema and salivary glands?

26. Why do the majority of doctors want to treat the symptoms of IC rather than the cause?

27. Why isn't the bacteria theory being looked at more closely? In the case of stomach ulcers, it took years and years for the medical community to finally admit ulcers were caused by bacteria.

28. Why do so many patients get IC from surgery? Is there anything being done about this?

29. Is any research being done on the White Blood Cell Count of IC patients?

30. Isn't there a better way to kill IC bacteria than taking antibiotics for 1 to 2 years straight and endangering the immune system?

31. Is there a study being done on the number of bad bacteria versus good bacteria among IC patients?

32. Is the eventual result of IC a wearing down our immune systems causing us to have other problems?

33. What is the connection between catheters and IC?

34. Is IC trauma to the bladder (surgery, intercourse, problems in the spine or anything that would affect normal bladder function) coupled with low immune resistance?

35. Why aren't all Urologist's using the broth culture (proven method) for bacteria identification?

36. Can DMSO force the bacteria deeper into the bladder wall? Can chlorpactin?

37. Is IC a result of the patient becoming resistant to antibiotics (like penicillin) in their lifetime?

38. I think something happened to each of us IC patients that permanently damaged our bladder walls. Now we have that weakness in our bladders and certain things that happen to our bodies make it flare-up. It can be one thing or it can be many different causes. That is why I think it is so hard to treat and get to the source of the cause of our flare-ups. We know what is going to happen during a flare-up but what causes it? Bacteria? yeast? Stress? Immune Weakness? Food Allergies? Yeast Buildup?

39. What is the connection between the spinal and pelvic floor muscles? Are microscopic amounts of blood in the urine connected to IC and if so why?
40. Is IC degenerative?
41. Are our immune systems attacking us? Are our immune systems over-reacting?

114. DO YOU LIVE IN AN AREA THAT IS CONDUCIVE TO MOLD GROWTH? I.E. DO YOU HAVE MOLD YOUR HOUSE OR YARD?
23 participants answered this last minute additional question. 78% answered Yes.

## A message from the questionnaire's author.

This questionnaire was created and compiled by Suzanne Bernhardt

**Silvrangel @AOL .COM**

It took me 4 months to create and compile this questionnaire. One cannot work so diligently on a project and not learn something from it. Below is my considered opinion of what I believe IC is for those interested.

Interstitial Cystitis patients have damaged or otherwise weak bladders resulting either from birth, hereditary factors, environmental pollutants (pesticides), excessive bladder infections or something else. This weakened bladder creates a ripe noncombative environment for bacteria. The bladder is too weak and/or damaged to fight off bacteria. The bacteria invading the bladders can come from surgery, sex, improper hygiene or from other parts of the body. Usually this invading type of destructive bacteria is not detected in normal lab cultures. Either because it is a different type of bacteria not commonly found in UTI's or because the bacteria has buried itself deep into the bladder walls. Not one factor but all factors exasperate yet are not the cause of Interstitial Cystitis. Bladder irritants can be chemical toxicity, environmental allergies (for example: mold), food allergies or sensitivities, body and food acids, stress, drugs, constipation, back problems, chlorine in drinking water, lack of oxygen to the pelvic region (from prolonged sitting) etc. Yeast/candida promotes the bacteria. The patient can take antibiotics to kill the bacteria once the proper antibiotic is matched to the particular invasive bacteria. However the initial problem is not being fixed. The bladder is still weak and/or damaged. Taking antibiotics long term may kill the invasive bacteria but it will also kill friendly bacteria and lower the immune function of the body. What needs to be done initially or simultaneously is to re-build the bladder to a normal functioning organ.

This can and should be done with vitamins, minerals, herbs, exercise, treatments like Aloe Vera or Elmiron and other measures yet untested or untried. Taking antibiotics alone will only solve half of the problem. The unrepaired bladder will continue to be approached and attacked by bacteria until it is repaired. Many people report feeling better while pregnant. This is also the healthiest of times for the IC patient. A time in which she is taking multi vitamin and mineral supplements while eating a balanced diet. Many patients complain of worsened symptoms prior to or directly after their menstrual periods or during ovulation. This may be due to hormone fluctuations acting as bladder irritants or increases in blood volume activating bacteria. The IC patient can either eliminate every single environmental toxin and irritant, or take antibiotics long term or rebuild the bladder through vitamin, minerals and herb therapy along with exercise. It is my opinion that short term antibiotic use along with aggressive bladder rebuilding therapy is the best solution.

Suzanne Bernhardt

The End

## I wish to thank the following participants

| | |
|---|---|
| AUBRY1025 | ROSE |
| BBRADY | BONNIE |
| BECKSPED | BECKY |
| CAM115 | ANGEL |
| CARAJEANT | DARLENE |
| CATH767 | CATHY |
| CCAT10 | JUDY |
| COWRU | LOIS |
| CRONEDTARR | DOREEN |
| CVERRILLI | CATHERINE |
| CYNGRAM | CYNTHIA |
| DAVID1201 | NANCY |
| DUTCHESS98 | AMY |
| EJACOBY739 | EVA |
| ERICHAR100 | KAREN |
| FANCTF3 | EDITH |
| FROBBINS | MARIANNE |
| GGELET | GLORIA |
| GIGGLEBIT | VICTORIA |
| GINNY1952 | GINNY |
| GOBSINCE | CAROLE |
| HICKS37 | KIM |
| HOOKERMF | MEGAN |
| HRLIE | TRACY |

| | |
|---|---|
| ICPAIN | BARBRA |
| JULESB40 | JULIE |
| KATCSR | KARA |
| KBATES1729 | KATRINA |
| KBURKIE | KELLY |
| LANDL30 | LINDSAY |
| LAURA3R | LAURA |
| LISAGART | LISA |
| LOEY | LOIS |
| LPSQ | JENNI |
| LSF16W | LORRIE |
| MALLEN3996 | MELYNN |
| MARJSGT | MARG |
| MBMACRAE | MONICA |
| MILOCASS | LORRAINE |
| MISIS | MELINDA |
| MODELMUSE | LESLIE |
| MSPEEBODY | JEANNE |
| NO SCREEN NAME | DEBORAH |
| NO SCREEN NAME | BARBARA |
| NO SCREEN NAME | SANDRA |
| NO SCREEN NAME | LOUISE |
| PBERN | PHYLLIS |
| PNIEB | NANCY |
| POISNFROG | BRENDA |
| PPC75PAUL | PAUL |
| RAMSHELL33 | SHELLEY |
| REE143G | MARIE |
| RELEASE22 | LINDA |
| RER25 | RENEE |
| RKACZM | JOANNE |
| SALLOH | SALLY |
| SANDYLHSOG | SANDY |
| SBARR29962 | SHIRLEY |
| SHARONDREW | SHARON |
| SILVRANGEL | SUZANNE |
| SKRISBERG | SANDI |
| SROBBIE123 | NO NAME GIVEN |
| SUSAN30305 | SUSAN |
| SWOLFSTAR | SANDY |
| TABRA1 | ANN |
| TPALMER301 | MARIANNE |
| TREKKINN | GAIL |
| WAS12201 | MARYANN |
| WEAVERCAT | NATASHA |
| ZORFIE | CAROLYN |
| ZUZER | DEBORAH |

Other books by Catherine M. Simone

## *Along the Healing Path*
### *Recovering from Interstitial Cystitis*
Copyright © 2000
ISBN: 0-9667750-1-5

## &

## *Awakening Through the Tears*
### *Interstitial Cystitis and*
### *The Mind/Body/Spirit Connection*
Copyright © 2002
ISBN: 0-9667750-2-3

To order call toll free 1-877-597-5766 or check with your local bookstore.

For more information, please visit http://www.ic-hope.com